What the Experts Say About Healthy Exchanges

"I find Ms. Lund's nutritional guidelines to be sound, and endorse her dietary recommendations when used in conjunction with traditional treatments and therapy."
                —Martin F. Koutcher, M.D.,
                Internal Medicine & Rheumatology Specialist,
                Methodist Hospital Division,
                Thomas Jefferson University Hospital

"JoAnna Lund's *The Arthritis Healthy Exchanges Cookbook* is an excellent publication. Dr. Sara Kramer's introduction gives one a very clear discussion and description of arthritis, which most people do not understand. The blend of a clear clinical description, the pathology of the disease, plus the importance of diet and exercise, along with medical management will be helpful to all. And the collection of recipes that are low in fat and rich in calcium will certainly help weight control. I will recommend this book to my patients without hesitation."
                —Richard Kreiter, M.D.,
                Orthopedist/Bone & Joint Specialist,
                Davenport, Iowa

ALSO BY JOANNA M. LUND

Healthy Exchanges Cookbook
HELP: The Healthy Exchanges Lifetime Plan
Cooking Healthy with a Man in Mind
Cooking Healthy with Kids in Mind
The Diabetic's Healthy Exchanges Cookbook
The Strong Bones Healthy Exchanges Cookbook
The Best of Healthy Exchanges Food Newsletter '92 Cookbook
Notes of Encouragement
Letters From the Heart
It's Not a Diet, It's a Way of Life (audiotape)

The Arthritis

Healthy

Exchanges

Cookbook

A HEALTHY EXCHANGES® COOKBOOK

JoAnna M. Lund

A Perigee Book

A Perigee Book
Published by The Berkley Publishing Group
A member of Penguin Putnam Inc.
200 Madison Avenue
New York, NY 10016

For more information about Healthy Exchanges products, contact:
Healthy Exchanges, Inc.
PO Box 124
DeWitt, IA 52742-0124
(319) 659-8234

First edition: May 1998

Published simultaneously in Canada.

The Penguin Putnam Inc. World Wide Web site address is
http://www.penguinputnam.com

Library of Congress Cataloging-in-Publication Data

Lund, JoAnna M.
    The arthritis healthy exchanges cookbook / by JoAnna M. Lund.
        p.   cm.
    "A healthy exchanges cookbook."
    "A Perigee book."
    Includes index.
    ISBN 0-399-52377-4
    1.   Arthritis—Diet therapy.   2.   Food exchange lists.   I.   Title.
    RC933.L86   1998   97-32731
    616.7'220654—dc21   CIP

Printed in the United States of America

10   9   8   7   6   5   4   3   2   1

As all my books are, this cookbook is dedicated in loving memory to my parents, Jerome and Agnes McAndrews. It is also dedicated to everyone who suffers from the pain of arthritis. Mom developed arthritis in her fifties, and each year the pain increased, to the point that just walking across the room caused her torment.

I hope that by sharing both my "common folk" healthy recipes and commonsense approach to healthy living, I can help you or your loved ones to avoid suffering in the same way. I also hope that many of these recipes become family favorites, to be enjoyed for years to come.

When faced with crippling arthritis, each of us may wonder, "Why me?" and not someone else. I know, because that's exactly what I did ten years ago, when I looked down at my hands and saw that they were beginning to become disfigured due to arthritis in my fingers. But, everything has a reason, and when I made better living choices, the effects of arthritis diminished. And when I changed my prayers to what I needed instead of what I wanted, my prayers were answered in ways I never could have imagined. No, the disfigurement didn't go away, but it also didn't get worse.

As usual, my mother had the appropriate poem for this book in her vast collection. The next time you are tempted to ask why, please read her words instead.

Thy Will Be Done

There are times "Thy Will Be Done"
    is hard to mean when we pray
Harder still to accept His Will, when
    we want our own way.
Prayers sometimes seem to go unheard
    when we ask for a request.
We feel lost and forsaken, forgetting that
    this could be a test.
No prayer goes unanswered, no tear is
    shed in vain.
No heart is broken without His
    comforting our pain.
If only we will trust Him completely,
    letting Him answer in His own way,
He will lift the cross we bear, and reveal to
    us the reason someday.
             —*Agnes Carrington McAndrews*

Contents

Acknowledgments

Never did I dream six years ago, when I began sharing my "common folk" healthy recipes and commonsense approach to healthy living, that I would touch so many lives in such positive ways. Nothing is done without the help of others, including sharing my recipes. For helping me so that I can share with so many others, I want to thank:

John Duff. He's been my first and only editor, but I can't imagine a better one in all of the publishing world.

Angela Miller and Coleen O'Shea. When I signed on with these "Big City" agents, I never dreamed they were such "country folk" at heart.

Phyllis Grann, Susan Petersen, Liz Perl, Barbara O'Shea, and everyone at Perigee Books. They all continue to encourage me to write from my heart as I compile my recipe books.

Rose Hoenig, R.D., L.D. No one compares to her when it comes to calculating diabetic exchanges and making sure my recipes are as accurate as can be in their nutrients.

Sara B. Kramer, M.D., F.A.C.R. She shares "real world" information on arthritis—no hype, no scare tactics, just common sense.

Shirley Morrow. When she typed my first recipe back in 1991, neither of us thought that she'd have to read my scribbling for well over 3,000 recipes (and the end still not in sight!).

Lori Hansen. Just as a painter can make the canvas come alive, she can make her computer "sing" as she calculates recipes.

Rita Ahlers. When she asked if she could help me in the kitchen, she never dreamed what lay ahead.

Barbara Alpert. It still amazes me how she has a way of organizing my words and getting out of me exactly what I mean.

Cliff Lund. If ever there was a better partner for me (both in marriage and business), I can't imagine who it would be!

God. He answered my prayers for help in His way, and with wonders I never thought possible.

Arthritis Pain and Recovery: My Own Story

Writing this cookbook has been a real emotional journey for me, because I know what it's like to suffer with arthritis pain. I know what it is to feel hopeless and out of control, and to be afraid that nothing you can do will help. This book doesn't promise any miracle cures, but it does provide suggestions on ways that nutrition may be able to ease your symptoms. So much research is ongoing into the many forms of arthritis, no one method will be right for everyone. Each individual's experience is different, but often we can learn from what helped someone else.

Here's my story.

The first time I knew I had arthritis, I was in my thirties and had hurt my back. The doctor did X-rays and found evidence that arthritis was setting in. After a year or two, my hands started hurting. I'll never forget the day I looked down and saw that both my middle fingers were starting to curve. I started crying when I realized that my fingers were no longer straight. In fact, I literally bawled having to confront the fact that my hands and feet were becoming deformed like my mother's had because of arthritis. At that time she could no longer hold a pen to write, open a jar, or grasp her eating utensils; she couldn't even wear the pretty shoes she loved anymore. I looked at her and I saw my own future—and it terrified me.

In my forties, I reached my all-time high weight of 300 pounds. My feet started bothering me, and I would wake up daily in pain. I could not walk on the flats of my feet but had to walk on the sides for at least ten minutes after I got out of bed. The combination of my weight and my arthritis was excruciating—there's just no other way to describe it.

Because my back would act up at the least little thing, I struggled to get through the day. My hands would hurt so bad, I couldn't open bottles or jars. And my feet—the pain made me wretched.

There wasn't much anyone could do for me. I took aspirin and tried to learn to live with it. One doctor gave me pills, a bottle of anti-inflammatory drugs, but when it ran out, I never refilled it. It didn't really work for me.

I also suffered from gout of the big toe (a form of arthritis), and had to take medication for it.

When I decided to quit dieting and change my focus to living a healthy lifestyle, I discovered a wonderful "side effect": the pain in my back, my hands, and my feet disappeared. I started eating a low-fat and low-sugar diet, and I made time in my day for moderate exercise. Without my realizing what was happening, the pain just disappeared.

I don't have the mobility in my hands I had when I was thirty, but what matters to me is that it hasn't deteriorated. In fact, in six years of healthy living, I've developed more strength. I don't have flare-up bouts of pain in my feet now, and I haven't had a backache since I lost 130 pounds. Now I jump out of bed every morning, work 14 to 16 hours on any given day, and when I go to bed, boom! I'm sound asleep.

I'm convinced there has to be a correlation between my healthy low-fat, low-sugar diet and the moderate exercise I do regularly. For me, what's worked best is walking, biking, and water aerobics. The walking is particularly meaningful to me. I can remember my mother having such terrible pain in her feet that my sisters and I used to take turns taking her to church. It was only a block and a half away from her apartment, but she was in too much pain to walk that little distance.

Getting started may seem tough, and if you haven't been doing much walking, your feet may hurt a little at first. Stick with it. Start by walking around the block or even just one side of it, then add a little bit more each time. Combined with losing weight and watching your diet, walking can be very helpful to anyone with arthritis.

The secret is doing what you can to remain limber. Riding a

bike is a good exercise for many people, but it can be stressful and difficult if you have bad knees. Water exercise is just about perfect for people with arthritis, because the water takes the weight off your joints and allows you to move.

One of the people who inspired me most when I was just starting out was a woman with severe arthritis at my local health club pool. She was there every day, doing whatever she could. I remember she called one exercise "milking the cow" (yes, it looks just like it sounds!) and said it helped her keep her hands limber.

Once I realized how good I was feeling, I did everything I could to sustain it. I also have arthritis in my upper shoulders, and occasionally, when I'm stressed by having too many deadlines to meet, I treat myself to a massage.

I also learned in my thirties how important it is to lift properly. Lift from your knees, not your back, the doctor taught me, and it became a good habit.

I was so determined to find a way to fight back against the pain and disability arthritis caused me. I didn't want my kids to have to take *me* to church. I loved my mother dearly but when her pain got so bad it hurt her to move, she made it very hard for those who loved her.

Positive attitude also plays an important role in coping with arthritis. By encouraging yourself to keep moving, to keep doing the best you can *the best you can,* you're more likely to succeed in making progress. Even if you can only sit in a chair and move your arms and legs, DO IT. Do something good for yourself, and your body will respond. Each day, try to do a little more.

It's a simple equation: The recipes in this book can help you work toward your goal of losing weight. Losing weight helps many people with arthritis. Carrying around less weight means less stress on your joints and more energy to do the things you want to do. And isn't that what life is all about, after all?

Introduction

Sara B. Kramer, M.D., F.A.C.R.

The word *arthritis* is defined simply as pain and swelling in a joint, but there are actually more than one hundred diseases considered forms of arthritis—and they affect forty million Americans. Some of these diseases have a basis in heredity, such as rheumatoid arthritis (RA) and lupus (also known as SLE, systemic lupus erythematosis). Some develop because of repeated or severe injuries to the body over time. Others have more to do with weakened bones due to osteoporosis or inadequate calcium.

In some kinds of arthritis, the disease is confined to the joint (osteoarthritis); in others, the disease may start in the joint but spread to other tissues or organs (rheumatoid arthritis). In some cases, arthritis is only part of the disease's manifestations (Lyme disease). And some forms of arthritis (including Reiter's disease and ankylosing spondylitis) may develop after a person is exposed to salmonella bacteria or chlamydia. These conditions may trigger the disease in individuals with certain hereditary factors, and even when the infection is gone, the arthritis remains.

How do you get from being a person with aches and pains to someone diagnosed with arthritis? A general rule is that if you're bothered by joint pain for more than a couple of weeks, or your pain is associated with fever or other symptoms, see your doctor. Everyone experiences joint pain and achy muscles sometimes—it's part of life—but if you're in constant discomfort and popping over-the-counter painkillers, you may have a more serious condition.

Your doctor will take a thorough medical history and may order blood tests and/or X-rays, in order to diagnose your condition. You may be referred to a rheumatologist, whose specialty is diseases of the joints and musculo-skeletal system. You may be tested for lupus or Lyme disease, depending on the symptoms you're experiencing.

Once you've been diagnosed, treatment may range from acetaminophen and other nonsteroidal anti-inflammatory drugs (NSAIDs) to stronger prescribed drugs. Whatever medication is prescribed, it's smart to ask questions and be certain you understand when to take it (on an empty stomach or with meals), and if there are any foods that should not be taken at the same time.

Let me give you a brief rundown of the three most common forms of arthritis:

Osteoarthritis

Whenever two bones meet, there is a joint. Healthy joints are covered with cartilage, a padding that absorbs the shock of the body's movement and also lessens friction. For those with osteoarthritis, the cartilage in the joints begins to wear away, eventually leading to bone rubbing against bone. Bone spurs may develop and press on nerves, causing pain. Bits of cartilage or bone may break off and "float" in the joint cavity. When bones with little or no padding rub together, you experience pain, often accompanied by inflammation. Common sites for osteoarthritis include weight-bearing joints (spine, hips, and knees); it's also common in fingers and in the spine. It can produce a loss of mobility or, at the least, stiffness in the body that encourages patients to move less and less.

The risk factors for osteoarthritis include trauma to the joint, obesity, overuse injuries (repetitive motions), congenital abnormalities (an easily dislocated joint, for example, like a shallow hip or shoulder socket), and heredity.

Sometimes surgery—from arthroscopic surgery to remove bits of bone and cartilage to joint replacement (hips and knees, most commonly)—is indicated.

Rheumatoid Arthritis

This common form of arthritis is considered an autoimmune disease, a type of disorder in which the body actually turns against itself. It strikes the joints of the fingers, wrists, feet, and ankles, and often hips and shoulders, causing pain, swelling, and stiffness. It's important that this disease be treated by a knowledgeable physician to minimize potential disability.

Gout

Gout is a metabolic disorder, a multi-metabolic disorder. It's the form of arthritis most sensitive to the foods you consume. Foods that are high in uric acid (purines) as well as alcohol can trigger gout attacks. Weight control is also important, because being overweight increases your body's production of uric acid.

Nutrition and Arthritis

Because there are so many different forms of arthritis, and because they have so many different causes, symptoms, and therapies, there is no one "diet prescription" that is right for every person with arthritis. The important thing to understand is that diet doesn't *cause* arthritis. A small number of people may have a specific food allergy, like milk or wheat or corn, that can produce an arthritis flare-up, but most do not.

There's been a lot of talk about "elimination" diets, which have you eliminate a suspect food from your diet for a week or more to try to determine if it's causing your symptoms. This can be a haphazard and even dangerous process to undertake on your own. By eliminating foods or groups of foods from your diet without firm evidence, you can end up with deficiencies. This is not to say that your observations aren't useful—they are. But you're better off working with a physician and dietitian to evaluate suspect foods; doing so on your own may produce inaccurate results and needlessly deprive your body of nutritious foods.

Instead, the emphasis should be on eating a well-balanced diet that encourages variety and moderation. Such a diet can help you feel your best, maintain your health, make you less likely to develop chronic diseases such as cancer and heart disease, and build a positive attitude when it comes to managing your arthritis.

What does it mean to eat a healthy diet?

- Vary your foods. This keeps you from getting bored and provides your body with all the nutrients it requires.

- Limit fat and cholesterol—think "moderation."

- Build your menus around fruit, vegetables, and grains.

- Emphasize foods low in sugar, salt, and sodium whenever possible.

- If you choose to drink alcohol, be aware of possible drug interactions and other potential concerns. (Alcohol combined with acetaminophen or methotrexate can damage the liver, for example). Alcohol can also definitely exacerbate gout. It's best to limit consumption to extreme moderation, maybe two glasses of wine a week. Also, for some individuals, the sulfites in many wines can produce arthritis flare-ups.

Weight Control and Arthritis

It's a simple fact: overweight people are more likely to have arthritis. If you're overweight, your risks for developing osteoarthritis in your weight-bearing joints as well as your hands are increased. Your knees are particularly endangered by having to support a greater than ideal weight for your height. As you get older, the closer you can remain to your best weight, the better chance you have to avoid developing problems.

If you're already overweight, you'll be happy to know that even a modest reduction in weight (about 10 pounds) also "trims" your risk of developing osteoarthritis.

But beware of how you approach the need to lose weight. The ongoing popularity of low-calorie weight-reduction diets, or diets that eliminate certain groups of foods, can actually be dangerous for anyone with arthritis symptoms. Maintaining the energy you need for an active life, as well as supporting the demands such activities make on your muscles and bones, requires eating a well-balanced, nutritious diet.

Remember, your goal is to protect the joints, not to drop pounds so quickly you won't be able to keep them off over time. You need enough calories to maintain a healthy weight, but not so many that you add unwanted pounds. A nutritious diet is a balanced diet, one that includes a variety of foods from each of the four basic food groups: meat, fish, and poultry; dairy; fruits and vegetables; breads, cereals, pasta, and rice. Think moderation—and think balance.

Meat, Fish, and Poultry. Many Americans eat more than a necessary amount of protein. You may be surprised to know that two servings daily for a total of 4 to 6 ounces is sufficient for most individuals. These protein servings deliver iron, the important B vitamins, and some minerals. Try to select low-fat products as often as you can. Best choices include white fish, water-packed tuna, swordfish, and chicken without the skin. Items with a medium fat content can also be part of a healthy diet and include lean ham, lamb, lean red meat (including lean ground beef). Trim visible fat off the lean meat you purchase, and try to limit egg yolks to no more than three per week.
Note: For some individuals, a diet that is substantially vegetarian has produced a lessening of symptoms. If you want to explore the possibility of a vegetarian diet, get help from a dietitian. You'll want to be certain to get all the protein you need from beans and soy foods, and you may need dietary supplements to assure your nutrient requirements are being met.

Dairy. Most adults require 2 to 3 servings daily from this group, which provides necessary calcium and consists of 1 cup of milk or yogurt, or 1 ounce of cheese. People with rheumatoid arthritis, especially women with RA, who are at greater risk of osteoporosis, may benefit from eating as many as 4 servings daily. Emphasize low-fat and nonfat dairy products to avoid developing high cholesterol.

* If you experience sensitivity to dairy products, discuss it with your doctor before skipping these foods; you may be a candidate for lactose-free products.

Fruits and Vegetables. To provide your body with vitamins A and C, fiber, and carbohydrates, at least 5 servings daily are recommended. Opt for variety—choose both yellow and dark-green leafy vegetables for vitamin A (The current RDA is 5,000 International Units [I.U.])—aim to get as much of this as you can from your diet; add a supplement if your physician advises it. Include citrus fruits as well as berries, peppers, and tomatoes for vitamin C (see chart below). Select fresh or frozen fruits rather than canned if possible, but choose those canned in juice over those canned in syrup. Canned vegetables generally have a high salt content, so they should be limited or possibly rinsed before use.
* A note here about what are called the **"nightshade vegetables"**: While there are no conclusive studies on the subject yet, many individual patients have reported some improvement or relief of symptoms by eliminating the foods in this group, which may cause a reaction in about one-fifth of arthritis cases. They include potatoes, tomatoes, eggplant, squash, and peppers. Red wine can produce a similar response. Let common sense prevail here. It's a good idea to avoid foods that make your pain worse, despite firm scientific evidence that they are not the cause.

Breads, Cereals, Pasta, Rice. This food group provides dietary fiber, iron, B vitamins, and minerals. Consume 5 to 6 servings per day from this group, avoiding baked goods that are high in fat and cereals with too much added sugar.

Other useful advice:

- Use salt and sodium in moderation. They can cause fluid retention and elevated blood pressure. Additionally, some medications (both nonsteroidal anti-inflammatory drugs and corticosteroids) cause the same problems. It's not enough to take the saltshaker off the table; most of our salt intake comes from processed and canned foods, so get in the habit of reading labels carefully.

- Bake or broil foods rather than frying. Use nonstick pans and low-cholesterol sprays instead of oils.

Good Sources of Vitamin C

(Many physicians recommend you get at least 1,000 mg/day, even though the current RDA is lower. Since C is a water-soluble vitamin, your body will flush out what it cannot use.)

Food	Vitamin C (mg)
1 guava	165
1 sweet red pepper	141
1 cup fresh-squeezed orange juice	124
1 cup cranberry juice cocktail	108
1 cup orange juice from concentrate	97
1 cup papaya	87
1 cup strawberries	85
1 cup grapefruit juice from concentrate	83
1 cup raw broccoli	82
1 kiwi	75
1 orange	70
1 cup cantaloupe cubes	68
1 sweet green pepper	66
1 mango	57
1 cup raw cauliflower	46
½ grapefruit	41

Some arthritis patients are sensitive to foods high in citrus. If you experience increased pain or inflammation after eating citrus, let your doctor know. Together you can decide if citrus should be limited or eliminated from your diet.

A Word about Water

Our bodies need water to survive. Water is the basis for the body's liquid lubricant of the joints, called synovial fluid. Many people who suffer from aches and pains are often also dehydrated. Hydrated cells simply work better, so make certain to drink water often throughout the day. Think of it as a "water prescription"— remember that it lubricates the joints! (Did you know—you're taller in the morning than later in the day because gravity actually squeezes water out of the body?)

I recommend that you drink at least six, and preferably eight or more, 8-ounce glasses of water each day. Water does everything from suppressing appetite (if your goal is losing weight) to flushing the by-products of your medication out of your system.

These nutrition guidelines are appropriate for just about anyone with arthritis. But people with gout may experience pain after eating foods containing high levels of a chemical called uric acid, which is produced by the breakdown of proteins by the body. Foods high in protein (particularly meats and dairy products) produce high levels of uric acid. When you have gout, your body accumulates uric acid. Although medication for gout does a good job of helping control symptoms, your doctor may advise you to adjust your diet in a way that lowers your uric acid levels. (Losing weight also helps!) Here's a chart that lists the foods highest in uric acid.

Foods with a High Uric Acid Content

Very High: organ meats, herring, herring roe, mussels, sardines, yeast

High: anchovies, bacon, codfish, goose, haddock, liver, kidneys, mackerel, salmon, scallops, trout, turkey, veal, venison

Moderately High: asparagus, bass, beef, bouillon, brains, chicken, crab, duck, eel, halibut, ham, kidney beans, lentils, lima beans, liverwurst, lobster, mushrooms, navy beans, oysters, peas, pork, rabbit, shrimp, spinach, tongue, tripe

If you have gout, these foods should be eaten in extreme moderation. If you have questions about including any of these foods in your diet, consult your physician.

What about Fish Oils?

Research has also suggested that the oils from certain cold-water fish may boost the immune system and help prevent some of the painful inflammation of rheumatoid arthritis. (These fish also provide excellent nutrition and are generally low in calories.) Here's a chart that lists the best food sources of these omega-3 fatty acids, but since the amounts needed to produce this anti-inflammatory effect may be substantial, it's better to consider supplementing your diet with these under a doctor's supervision.

Be careful, though. You *can* take in too much fish oil (which has a blood-thinning effect), especially if you take fish-oil capsules as a supplement. Consult your doctor for more information about whether omega-3 could be right for you. There are no long-term studies yet about the effects of this supplement.

Atlantic salmon	Atlantic mackerel
Anchovies, canned in oil, drained	Bluefin tuna (raw, as in sushi or sashimi)
Atlantic herring	Rainbow trout
Sablefish	Atlantic sardines, canned in oil, drained
Chinook salmon	
Whitefish	Bluefish
Canned pink salmon	Rainbow smelt
Atlantic pickled herring	White (albacore) tuna, canned in water
Swordfish	

Arthritis Drugs and Vitamins—
What Should You Know?

Some of the drugs prescribed for arthritis symptoms may deplete the body of certain necessary nutrients. (Corticosteroids and NSAIDs, for instance, can cause fluid retention and even high blood pressure.) Some can irritate and cause ulcers, or affect the liver. Others may interact with an over-the-counter headache tablet or even a vitamin supplement.

While a multivitamin is recommended for just about every arthritis patient, you should always check with your doctor before taking additional supplements beyond the Recommended Daily Allowance (RDA). Excesses of nutrients, even ones that are supposed to be healthy, can hurt you. For example, too much Vitamin C, taken in pill form, can potentially cause ulcers because it's an acid—ascorbic acid. (Don't let this discourage you from eating fruits and veggies high in vitamin C—it's much less likely to happen with food.)

Antioxidants. Some studies have suggested that people with osteoarthritis often have very low levels of antioxidant nutrients, such as vitamin E, beta-carotene, and selenium, and by choosing foods that contain them (and sometimes taking supplements when advised by a physician) can help neutralize some of the free radicals released during joint inflammation.

Folic Acid. Some patients, especially those with rheumatoid arthritis, may be prescribed a drug called methotrexate, which interferes with the body's absorption of folic acid. In most cases, your physician will advise a supplement. You'll usually get the recommended daily allowance of folic acid (400 micrograms) in a multivitamin, or in a serving of Product 19 or Total cereals. Beans are also good sources of folic acid. Currently, some studies are reviewing the effects of taking B-12 and folic acid together, and have reported some improvement in patients taking these supplements.

Calcium. If you don't get enough calcium in your diet, you're already at risk for developing osteoporosis. Without sufficient amounts of this important nutrient, your bones may become thin and brittle, so it's important to get 1,000 to 1,500 mg calcium per day. It's also vital to get enough vitamin D so you can absorb the calcium in your diet. Always look for fortified dairy products, and get enough sunlight (a problem for many older women).

Some of the medications prescribed for arthritis symptoms (steroids, corticosteroids, methotrexate, cyclosporin) block calcium absorption and can actually cause osteoporosis. If you're being treated with any of those, it's extra-important to keep your calcium up. And if you have other risk factors for osteoarthritis, ask to get monitored for bone density. Patients taking these drugs should also be careful to limit sodium, since water retention is not uncommon.

An interesting link between osteoporosis and arthritis is currently being researched. Patients at risk for osteoporosis who opt for estrogen replacement therapy may be protecting themselves from developing arthritis symptoms.

Iron. Iron is necessary for good health, and many women don't get enough iron from the foods they eat. But excess iron can cause a problem for arthritis patients, as it's been linked to inflammation. You can develop a kind of arthritis called hemachromatosis caused by absorbing too much iron. Again, your best bet is to check with your physician and have your iron monitored.

Arthritis and Exercise

Exercise is always part of my prescription to my patients with arthritis. This disease can have a devastating effect on range of motion—your ability to stretch and reach, to bend and straighten—and also on the amount of muscle you have. Exercise helps you overcome stiffness and keep your joints moving; it maintains muscle tone and builds muscle around joints, which helps support those joints; it helps prevent osteoporosis; it strengthens the heart; it burns calories for weight control; and it gives you a strong sense of well-being.

But exercise doesn't have to be complicated. It can be as simple as going for a walk regularly, just to keep the body moving.

Don't worry about your pace or whether you're working hard enough when you lace on a pair of supportive walking shoes and stroll around your neighborhood or mall. As the shoe ad says, just do it.

But don't let your enthusiasm drive you to do too much too quickly. Build up slowly, so your joints and muscles have a chance to get accustomed to what you're asking of them. Start with a few blocks, or just one if that's all you can manage slowly. Remember that you can't "cram" for exercise. You'll feel better and get better results when you take time off to rest your body. Work muscles on alternate days; that way, they can heal and strengthen and get more out of the next workout. Bodybuilders know this and usually work upper body on alternate days to lower body.

If you're in shape to jog or run, go ahead and do it—in moderation. When millions of Americans began jogging a few years ago, some studies indicated that runners ought to worry about developing premature arthritis from such a "high-impact" sport. But further research was more encouraging, and unless you experience a serious injury or bad fall, the benefits of running outweigh the worries.

If you do get an injury, stop what you're doing. Rest the injured part and ice it to prevent swelling. During your recovery, you don't have to lose the aerobic fitness you've developed. Simply move your workout into the pool.

Water exercise is a natural for anyone with arthritis. Exercises you may struggle to do on land feel relaxed and easy in a warm water environment. If you're not a swimmer, join an aqua aerobics or deep-water running class at a local pool.

I also encourage my patients to include strength training—lifting light weights on a regular basis. This is especially important for women at risk of developing osteoporosis, but it's good for men and women of all ages. There are books and videos to provide instruction, and the Arthritis Foundation offers a videotape called PACE (People with Arthritis Can Exercise).

Do all you can to avoid injuries. Sports injuries (smashed-up knees from contact sports, for example) can often lead to osteoarthritis as you age. This is another reason why wearing protective gear is so important, especially in sports like Roller-blading.

Lifestyle Changes Can Make a Difference

Okay—once you've focused on nutrition and exercise, what else can you do to cope with your arthritis? My best advice: DE-STRESS!

Eliminating as many sources of stress in your life as you can is an excellent and worthwhile tactic. You may decide to consider a less stressful job, or that your commute is too demanding. Too drastic? Well, what about the workplace itself? Is your desk or work station the appropriate height? Are your computer and mouse in the right place? If they're not, you're likely to experience overuse and repetitive stress syndromes. Make sure you have a proper chair and that you sit in the chair correctly. (Sit back in your chair, not on the edge as so many of us do.) Remember to get up and move around frequently. Practice stretching exercises at your desk, and gently twist and release your torso so your back doesn't tighten up, especially your upper back.

It's essential to get adequate rest, especially if you have rheumatoid arthritis. Take a nap in the afternoon or early evening without feeling guilty about it—it's good for you. When you're preparing meals, take rest breaks as needed. Arrange your kitchen so the items you use most often are easily available, either on the counter or in accessible cabinets. Use convenience foods to make food prep simpler and faster; trade in your hand-cranked can opener for an electric one.

The ultimate best de-stresser: take an active approach to your life. Take charge of making your life work better for you. The Arthritis Foundation offers self-help courses, warm-water exercise classes, and support groups to help patients handle the stresses of their lives and conditions. There are chapters in every state and they're a great source of information, referrals, and courses. (Call 1-800-283-7800 for information.)

What's New—Now

It seems that every year you read about new research that finally offers a "cure" to people in pain, but it's important to use care in trying these new therapies. Just because a product is widely available and advertised in drugstores doesn't mean it's been properly tested and approved for use. Take an active role in learning what may be new or recently available, but get your physician's okay before you "swallow" what they're selling!

Glucosamine and Chondroitin Sulfate. There's been a lot of attention given to the effect of supplements of glucosamine and chondroitin sulfates on osteoarthritis (which causes a gradual erosion of the cartilage that cushions the tips of bones). These substances are naturally found in joints, where they promote the synthesis and repair of collagen. Some studies have produced encouraging results, suggesting that supplements of these "building blocks" of joint cartilage can actually slow, halt, or even prevent the degeneration of cartilage as you age. More research needs to be done before these supplements are considered a prescribed treatment, but stay tuned. Glucosamine has been prescribed in Europe for some time to decrease pain and increase mobility, but because no pharmaceutical company owns rights to the product, research in the United States has been minimal.

Capsaicin. Some physicians have offered their patients a topical cream called capsaicin, which is the main ingredient in chile peppers. It contains a chemical that inhibits substance P, a compound that breaks down the cartilage in people with osteoarthritis. In one study at the University of Miami School of Medicine, a number of people noted greater flexibility after using this cream, which does have an uncomfortable side effect—a mild to intense skin burning sensation. Be careful if you decide to try topical rubs at the suggestion of your physician—they can actually burn the skin without your realizing it because they also have a numbing effect.

Some claims for cures or new diets are health frauds with no scientific basis for the claims. Some are still under study. And some have never been reviewed by scientists for viability and safety. It's important to remain hopeful for a cure or treatment to prevent or heal the disabling injuries of arthritis. But don't let your desire for such a medical "miracle" lead you to take chances with your health.

You're in Charge Here

Whatever form of arthritis you have, you can live an active and full life by following these simple guidelines:

Control your weight. By staying as close as you can to a recommended weight, you reduce the stress on joints like knees and hips.

Conserve energy. Get all the rest you need so you don't suffer from fatigue, and avoid overusing joints that are already stressed by your illness.

Get regular exercise. It can make you feel less anxious about your condition and also ease the pain of your joints and muscles by ensuring a fuller range of motion.

In most cases, arthritis is a chronic disease. Because of that, it requires a different approach than an acute condition. It means learning to live as well as you can *with* your disease. Your initial reaction at diagnosis may be to ask "Why me?" You may even experience depression or a feeling of hopelessness. Try hard not to give in to it! Instead, take an active approach to coping with your arthritis:

- Learn all you can about your disease, and be involved in your treatment.

- Develop a good working relationship with your physician.

- Consider changes in your career or lifestyle that may help you handle the stress of your condition.

- Create a support system of family and friends who will be there for you.

- Most of all, choose to be optimistic. A positive attitude can be the best medicine!

Gin and Raisins

I'd like you to meet Bill Wundram, daily columnist for the *Quad-City Times* for the past fifteen or so years and an award-winning journalist who's been a great friend to me and to Healthy Exchanges. When I first read the story he's about to share with you, I smiled from ear to ear. Most of us who've suffered with some form of arthritis hope that scientists will someday find a cure. (For now, we'll do the best we can through nutrition, exercise, and whatever else our doctors may prescribe.) But sometimes what's known as "folk medicine" can provide some respite from our symptoms. At the very least, this story is a prescription for laughter, which may help you feel better already!

Gin and Raisins

by Bill Wundram
(based on columns originally published in March 1994)

I have been accused of always writing about home remedies such as warm goose grease for chest colds and Sloan's liniment and sugar for sore throat. In my wanderings, I have encountered any number of successful kitchen ointments, but what follows—gin and raisins—may be the most widely publicized of our time.

"It is the craziest thing," says Al Hallene, Sr., of Moline, Illinois, the president of Montgomery Elevator International, who may have been the one who first started spreading the word of this "curative" process to the afflicted millions. Then Paul Harvey of *The Rest of the Story* fame, began talking about it on the airwaves, and it's since been repeated at every crossroads junction general store and at every bridge club. It has become the nation's celebrated "gin and raisin" cure for arthritis, and it appears to have originated right here in Quad-Cities USA, growing healthier every day.

Let's start at the beginning. Hallene said he and a Moline dentist were golfing. The dentist complained of a slight arthritis in his hand. Hallene offered sympathy and said he had the same thing. They both had heard about a strange "gin and raisin" recipe for relief. It was said to come, not from a rattle-shaking witch doctor but by way of a physician in the eastern United States. In Hallene's words, "Arthritis is a shifty thing, so it's difficult to say if it works or not."

Well, what is it? Here's the formula: Buy a box of golden raisins and spread them out in a glass pie plate. Not a tin pie plate but a glass pie plate. Plastic might work but glass is best. Then, go someplace where they sell booze. Buy a fifth of the cheapest gin. I called Gendler's Wine Cellar in Rock Island for the name of a good, inexpensive brand and the attendant instantly said, "Aha, the gin and raisin cure." He sure did know what I was talking about before I even began to talk. Well, at the lower-priced end of the scale, he suggested Gordon's or Gilbey's gin. You take this gin and pour it onto the golden raisins scattered in the pie pan. You let the whole works marinate for exactly seven days. After a week, the raisins have absorbed all the gin. No gin should be left. Those raisins are bloated like Iowa pigs at the slop trough. Now, the fun begins, if you have arthritis. You eat nine of those gin-sated raisins a day. There will be a lot of them, so you better seal them in a jar so they don't dry out. If you're lucky, by the time you are finished with all the raisins, your arthritis pain may be relieved.

This celebrated "gin and raisin" cure came to attention during a meeting of the highly respected MacArthur Foundation in Chicago. Hallene is a director of this organization (which gives out the "genius" awards), likely the most philanthropic group in America and one of the great benefactors of PBS. One board member was severely afflicted with arthritis, and Hallene casually mentioned that, as a long shot, he might try the "gin and raisin" treatment. At the time, this particular director could barely shake hands. At the next meeting, his condition was notably improved. "Say, that stuff really works," he said, congratulating Hallene. Across the table that day was Paul Harvey, the noted broadcaster, who is also a director of the MacArthur Foundation. "Paul Harvey's rabbit ears flopped up, and it wasn't long before he had the arthritis formula of gin and raisins on the air," says Hallene. Hallene was credited, and the recipe went out to millions of listeners.

After my original column ran, the paper received a lot of mail on the subject. I learned that the recipe is nothing new. It goes back to 1625, and is something the Germans have known all along. Waltraud Martens of Davenport, Iowa, told me Germans have been mixing raisins and schnapps (or any form of grain liquor) for years to cure all that ails them, not just arthritis.

A lady from Toledo, Ohio, published her story in a church bulletin. She began eating nine raisins a day on October 10 and saw results in just a few weeks. She wrote, "Why does this recipe bring such fantastic results? As far back as biblical times, people of India and Egypt discovered the healing powers of juniper berries. Gin is made from natural grains and juniper berries . . . I, who cannot stand the odor of alcoholic beverages and limit my alcohol content to the swallow of communion wine, am now telling everyone about gin-soaked raisins. I'm firmly 'hooked' on this weird remedy." She added that it was also important to keep those arms and legs moving.

There is more. At one meeting of the foundation, a director said that he wasn't sure if he was to eat nine raisins a day or drink nine shots of gin a day, so he did both, and has never felt better. "The 'gin and raisin' thing has given relief to some people around Montgomery Elevator who have arthritis problems," Hallene notes. "It's either something of an answer, or the greatest placebo."

About the Author: Bill Wundram has been writing, he says, "since the lava dried." His column appears seven days a week in the *Quad-City Times*, he's been named a master columnist by the Iowa Press Association and, he adds, "Doing a daily column either keeps me out of the taverns or puts me in them. I tell my wife that I'm good to her. I'm gone a lot." He's written just about all there is to write, "from pig kissing and frying of eggs on sidewalks to shopping all day for orange slices with Red Skelton and bumming a ride with Bob Hope, to covering the pope and scouring the Midwest to find the best pork tenderloin sandwich."

Dear Friends,

People often ask me why I include the same general information at the beginning of all my cookbooks. If you've seen any of my other books, you'll know that my "common folk" recipes are just one part of the Healthy Exchanges picture. You know that I firmly believe—and say so whenever and wherever I can—that *Healthy Exchanges is not a diet, it's a way of life!* That's why I include the story of Healthy Exchanges in every book, because I know that the tale of my struggle to lose weight and regain my health is one that speaks to the hearts of many thousands of people. And because Healthy Exchanges is not just a collection of recipes, I always include the wisdom that I've learned from my own experiences and the knowledge of the health and cooking professionals I meet. Whether it's learning about nutrition or making shopping and cooking easier, no Healthy Exchanges book would be complete without features like "A Peek into My Pantry" or "JoAnna's Ten Commandments of Successful Cooking."

Even if you've read my other books, you still might want to skim the following chapters—you never know when I'll slip in a new bit of wisdom or suggest a new product that will make your journey to health an easier and tastier one. If you're sharing this book with a friend or family member, you'll want to make sure they read the following pages before they start stirring up the recipes.

If this is the first book of mine that you've read, I want to welcome you with all my heart to the Healthy Exchanges Family. (And, of course, I'd love to hear your comments or questions. See the back of this book for my mailing address . . . or come visit if you happen to find yourself in DeWitt, Iowa—just ask anybody for directions to Healthy Exchanges!)

Jo Anna

JoAnna M. Lund

and Healthy

Exchanges®

Food is the first invited guest to every special occasion in every family's memory scrapbook. From baptism to graduation, from weddings to wakes, food brings us together.

It wasn't always that way at our house. I used to eat alone, even when my family was there, because while they were dining on real food, I was nibbling at whatever my newest diet called for. In fact, for twenty-eight years, I called myself the diet queen of DeWitt, Iowa.

I tried every diet I ever came across, every one I could afford, and every one that found its way to my small town in eastern Iowa. I was willing to try anything that promised to "melt off the pounds," determined to deprive my body in every possible way in order to become thin at last.

I sent away for expensive "miracle" diet pills. I starved myself on the Cambridge Diet and the Bahama Diet. I gobbled diet candies, took thyroid pills, fiber pills, prescription and over-the-counter diet pills. I went to endless weight-loss support group meetings—but I somehow managed to turn healthy programs such as Overeaters Anonymous, Weight Watchers, and TOPS into unhealthy diets . . . diets I could never follow for more than a few months.

I was determined to discover something that worked long-term, but each new failure increased my desperation that I'd never find it.

I ate strange concoctions and rubbed on even stranger potions.

I tried liquid diets. I agreed to be hypnotized. I tried reflexology and even had an acupressure device stuck in my ear!

Does my story sound a lot like yours? I'm not surprised. No wonder the weight-loss business is a billion-dollar industry!

Every new thing I tried seemed to work—at least at first. And losing that first five or ten pounds would get me so excited, I'd believe that this new miracle diet would, finally, get my weight off for keeps.

Inevitably, though, the initial excitement wore off. The diet's routine and boredom set in, and I quit. I shoved the pills to the back of the medicine chest; pushed the cans of powdered shake mix to the rear of the kitchen cabinets; slid all the program materials out of sight under my bed; and once more I felt like a failure.

Like most dieters, I quickly gained back the weight I'd lost each time, along with a few extra "souvenir" pounds that seemed always to settle around my hips. I'd done the diet-lose-weight-gain-it-all-back "yo-yo" on the average of once a year. It's no exaggeration to say that over the years I've lost 1,000 pounds—and gained back 1,150 pounds.

Finally, at the age of forty-six I weighed more than I'd ever imagined possible. I'd stopped believing that any diet could work for me. I drowned my sorrows in sacks of cake donuts and wondered if I'd live long enough to watch my grandchildren grow up.

Something had to change.

I had to change.

Finally, I did.

I'm just over fifty now—and I'm 130 pounds less than my all-time high of close to 300 pounds. I've kept the weight off for more than six years. I'd like to lose another ten pounds, but I'm not obsessed about it. If it takes me two or three years to accomplish it, that's okay.

What I *do* care about is never saying hello again to any of those unwanted pounds I said good-bye to!

How did I jump off the roller coaster I was on? For one thing, I finally stopped looking to food to solve my emotional problems. But what really shook me up—and got me started on the path that changed my life—was Operation Desert Storm in early 1991. I sent three children off to the Persian Gulf War—my son-in-law Matt, a medic in Special Forces; my daughter Becky, a full-time college student and member of a medical unit in the Army Reserve; and my son James, a member of the Inactive Army Reserve reactivated as a chemicals expert.

Somehow, knowing that my children were putting their lives on the line got me thinking about my own mortality—and I knew in my heart the last thing they needed while they were overseas was to get a letter from home saying that their mother was ill because of a food-related problem.

The day I drove the third child to the airport to leave for Saudi Arabia, something happened to me that would change my life for the better—and forever. I stopped praying my constant prayer as a professional dieter, which was simply "Please, God, let me lose ten pounds by Friday." Instead, I began praying, "God, please help me not to be a burden to my kids and my family." I quit praying for what I wanted and started praying for what I needed— and in the process my prayers were answered. I couldn't keep the kids safe—that was out of my hands—but I could try to get healthier to better handle the stress of it. It was the least I could do on the homefront.

That quiet prayer was the beginning of the new JoAnna Lund. My initial goal was not to lose weight or create healthy recipes. I only wanted to become healthier for my kids, my husband, and myself.

Each of my children returned safely from the Persian Gulf War. But something didn't come back—the 130 extra pounds I'd been lugging around for far too long. I'd finally accepted the truth after all those agonizing years of suffering through on-again, off-again dieting.

There are no "magic" cures in life.

No "miracle" potion, pill, or diet will make unwanted pounds disappear.

I found something better than magic, if you can believe it. When I turned my weight and health dilemma over to God for guidance, a new JoAnna Lund and Healthy Exchanges were born.

I discovered a new way to live my life—and uncovered an unexpected talent for creating easy "common folk" healthy recipes, and sharing my commonsense approach to healthy living. I learned that I could motivate others to change their lives and adopt a positive outlook. I began publishing cookbooks and a monthly food newsletter, and speaking to groups all over the country.

I like to say, *"When life handed me a lemon, not only did I make healthy, tasty lemonade, I wrote the recipe down!"*

What I finally found was not a quick fix or a short-term diet, but a great way to live well for a lifetime.

I want to share it with you.

Food Exchanges and Weight Loss Choices™

If you've ever been on one of the national weight-loss programs like Weight Watchers or Diet Center, you've already been introduced to the concept of measured portions of different food groups that make up your daily food plan. If you are not familiar with such a system of weight-loss choices or exchanges, here's a brief explanation. (If you want or need more detailed information, you can write to the American Dietetic Association or the American Diabetes Association for comprehensive explanations.)

The idea of food exchanges is to divide foods into basic food groups. The foods in each group are measured in servings that have comparable values. These groups include Proteins/Meats, Breads/Starches, Vegetables, Fats, Fruits, Skim Milk, Free Foods, and Optional Calories.

Each choice or exchange included in a particular group has about the same number of calories and a similar carbohydrate, protein, and fat content as the other foods in that group. Because any food on a particular list can be "exchanged" for any other food in that group, it makes sense to call the food groups *exchanges* or *choices*.

I like to think we are also "exchanging" bad habits and food choices for good ones!

By using Weight Loss Choices or exchanges you can choose from a variety of foods without having to calculate the nutrient value of each one. This makes it easier to include a wide variety of foods in your daily menus and gives you the opportunity to tailor your choices to your unique appetite.

If you want to lose weight, you should consult your physician or other weight-control expert regarding the number of servings that would be best for you from each food group. Since men generally require more calories than women, and since the requirements for growing children and teenagers differ from those of adults, the right number of exchanges for any one person is a personal decision.

I have included a suggested plan of weight-loss choices in the pages following the exchange lists. It's a program I used to lose 130 pounds, and it's the one I still follow today.

(If you are a diabetic or have been diagnosed with heart problems, it is best to meet with your physician before using this or any other food program or recipe collection.)

Food Group Weight Loss Choices/Exchanges

Not all food group exchanges are alike. The ones that follow are for anyone who's interested in weight loss or maintenance. If you are a diabetic, you should check with your health-care provider or dietitian to get the information you need to help you plan your diet. Diabetic exchanges are calculated by the American Diabetic Association, and information about them is provided in *The Diabetic's Healthy Exchanges Cookbook* (Perigee Books).

Every Healthy Exchanges recipe provides calculations in three ways:

- Weight Loss Choices/Exchanges

- Calories, Fat, Protein, Carbohydrates, and Fiber Grams, and Sodium in milligrams

- Diabetic Exchanges calculated for me by a Registered Dietitian

Healthy Exchanges recipes can help you eat well and recover your health, whatever your health concerns may be. Please take a few minutes to review the exchange lists and the suggestions that follow on how to count them. You have lots of great eating in store for you!

Proteins

Meat, poultry, seafood, eggs, cheese, and legumes. One exchange of Protein is approximately 60 calories. Examples of one Protein choice or exchange:

> 1 ounce cooked weight of lean meat, poultry, or seafood
> 2 ounces white fish
> 1½ ounces 97% fat-free ham
> 1 egg (limit to no more than 4 per week)
> ¼ cup egg substitute
> 3 egg whites
> ¾ ounce reduced-fat cheese
> ½ cup fat-free cottage cheese
> 2 ounces cooked or ¾ ounce uncooked dry beans
> 1 tablespoon peanut butter (also count 1 fat exchange)

Breads

Breads, crackers, cereals, grains, and starchy vegetables. One exchange of Bread is approximately 80 calories. Examples of one Bread choice or exchange:

> 1 slice bread or 2 slices reduced-calorie bread (40 calories or less)
> 1 roll, any type (1 ounce)
> ½ cup cooked pasta or ¾ ounce uncooked (scant ½ cup)
> ½ cup cooked rice or 1 ounce uncooked (⅓ cup)
> 3 tablespoons flour
> ¾ ounce cold cereal
> ½ cup cooked hot cereal or ¾ ounce uncooked (2 tablespoons)
> ½ cup corn (kernels or cream-style) or peas
> 4 ounces white potato, cooked, or 5 ounces uncooked
> 3 ounces sweet potato, cooked, or 4 ounces uncooked
> 3 cups air-popped popcorn
> 7 fat-free crackers (¾ ounce)
> 3 (2½-inch squares) graham crackers

2 (3/4-ounce) rice cakes or 6 mini
1 tortilla, any type (6-inch diameter)

Fruits

All fruits and fruit juices. One exchange of Fruit is approximately 60 calories. Examples of one Fruit choice or exchange:

1 small apple or 1/2 cup slices
1 small orange
1/2 medium banana
3/4 cup berries (except strawberries and cranberries)
1 cup strawberries or cranberries
1/2 cup canned fruit, packed in fruit juice or rinsed well
2 tablespoons raisins
1 tablespoon spreadable fruit spread
1/2 cup apple juice (4 fluid ounces)
1/2 cup orange juice (4 fluid ounces)
1/2 cup applesauce

Skim Milk

Milk, buttermilk, and yogurt. One exchange of Skim Milk is approximately 90 calories. Examples of one Skim Milk choice or exchange:

1 cup skim milk
1/2 cup evaporated skim milk
1 cup low-fat buttermilk
3/4 cup plain fat-free yogurt
1/3 cup nonfat dry milk powder

Vegetables

All fresh, canned, or frozen vegetables other than the starchy vegetables. One exchange of Vegetable is approximately 30 calories. Examples of one Vegetable choice or exchange:

1/2 cup vegetable
1/4 cup tomato sauce
1 medium fresh tomato
1/2 cup vegetable juice

Fats

Margarine, mayonnaise, vegetable oils, salad dressings, olives, and nuts. One exchange of fat is approximately 40 calories. Examples of one Fat choice or exchange:

> *1 teaspoon margarine or 2 teaspoons reduced-calorie margarine*
> *1 teaspoon butter*
> *1 teaspoon vegetable oil*
> *1 teaspoon mayonnaise or 2 teaspoons reduced-calorie mayonnaise*
> *1 teaspoon peanut butter*
> *1 ounce olives*
> *¼ ounce pecans or walnuts*

Free Foods

Foods that do not provide nutritional value but are used to enhance the taste of foods are included in the Free Foods group. Examples of these are spices, herbs, extracts, vinegar, lemon juice, mustard, Worcestershire sauce, and soy sauce. Cooking sprays and artificial sweeteners used in moderation are also included in this group. However, you'll see that I include the caloric value of artificial sweeteners in the Optional Calories of the recipes.

You may occasionally see a recipe that lists "free food" as part of the portion. According to the published exchange lists, a free food contains fewer than 20 calories per serving. Two or three servings per day of free foods/drinks are usually allowed in a meal plan.

Optional Calories

Foods that do not fit into any other group but are used in moderation in recipes are included in Optional Calories. Foods that are counted in this way include sugar-free gelatin and puddings, fat-free mayonnaise and dressings, reduced-calorie whipped toppings, reduced-calorie syrups and jams, chocolate chips, coconut, and canned broth.

Sliders™

These are 80 Optional Calorie increments that do not fit into any particular category. You can choose which food group to *slide* these into. It is wise to limit this selection to approximately three to four per day to ensure the best possible nutrition for your body while still enjoying an occasional treat.

Sliders may be used in either of the following ways:

1. If you have consumed all your Protein, Bread, Fruit, or Skim Milk Weight Loss Choices for the day, and you want to eat additional foods from those food groups, you simply use a Slider. It's what I call "healthy horse trading." Remember that Sliders may not be traded for choices in the Vegetables or Fats food groups.

2. Sliders may also be deducted from your Optional Calories for the day or week. ¼ Slider equals 20 Optional Calories; ½ Slider equals 40 Optional Calories; ¾ Slider equals 60 Optional Calories; and 1 Slider equals 80 Optional Calories.

Healthy Exchanges Weight Loss Choices

My original Healthy Exchanges program of Weight Loss Choices was based on an average daily total of 1,400 to 1,600 calories per day. That was what I determined was right for my needs, and for those of most women. Because men require additional calories (about 1,600 to 1,900), here are my suggested plans for women and men. *(If you require more or fewer calories, please revise this plan to meet your individual needs.)*

Each day, women should plan to eat:

2 Skim Milk servings, 90 calories each
2 Fat servings, 40 calories each
3 Fruit servings, 60 calories each
4 Vegetable servings or more, 30 calories each
5 Protein servings, 60 calories each
5 Bread servings, 80 calories each

Each day, men should plan to eat:

2 *Skim Milk servings, 90 calories each*
4 *Fat servings, 40 calories each*
3 *Fruit servings, 60 calories each*
4 *Vegetable servings or more, 30 calories each*
6 *Protein servings, 60 calories each*
7 *Bread servings, 80 calories each*

Young people should follow the program for Men but add 1 Skim Milk serving for a total of 3 servings.

You may also choose to add up to 100 Optional Calories per day, and up to 21 to 28 Sliders per week at 80 calories each. If you choose to include more Sliders in your daily or weekly totals, deduct those 80 calories from your Optional Calorie "bank."

A word about **Sliders**: These are to be counted toward your totals after you have used your allotment of choices of Skim Milk, Protein, Bread, and Fruit for the day. By "sliding" an additional choice into one of these groups, you can meet your individual needs for that day. Sliders are especially helpful when traveling, stressed-out, eating out, or for special events. I often use mine so I can enjoy my favorite Healthy Exchanges desserts. Vegetables are not to be counted as Sliders. Enjoy as many Vegetable Choices as you need to feel satisfied. Because we want to limit our fat intake to moderate amounts, additional Fat Choices should not be counted as Sliders. If you choose to include more fat on an *occasional* basis, count the extra choices as Optional Calories.

Keep a daily food diary of your Weight Loss Choices, checking off what you eat as you go. If, at the end of the day, your required selections are not 100 percent accounted for, but you have done the best you can, go to bed with a clear conscience. There will be days when you have ¼ Fruit or ½ Bread left over. What are you going to do—eat two slices of an orange or half a slice of bread and throw the rest out? I always say, "Nothing in life comes out exact." Just do the best you can . . . *the best you can.*

Try to drink at least eight 8-ounce glasses of water a day. Water truly is the "nectar" of good health.

As a little added insurance, I take a multivitamin each day. It's not essential, but if my day's worth of well-planned meals "bites the dust" when unexpected events intrude on my regular routine, my body still gets its vital nutrients.

The calories listed in each group of Choices are averages. Some choices within each group may be higher or lower, so it's important to select a variety of different foods instead of eating the same three or four all the time.

Use your Optional Calories! They are what I call "life's little extras." They make all the difference in how you enjoy your food and appreciate the variety available to you. Yes, we can get by without them, but do you really want to? Keep in mind that you should be using all your daily Weight Loss Choices first to ensure you are getting the basics of good nutrition. But I guarantee that Optional Calories will keep you from feeling deprived—and help you reach your weight-loss goals.

Sodium, Fat, Cholesterol, and Processed Foods

A *re Healthy Exchanges ingredients really healthy?*

When I first created Healthy Exchanges, many people asked about sodium, about whether it was necessary to calculate the percentage of fat, saturated fat, and cholesterol in a healthy diet, and about my use of processed foods in many recipes. I researched these questions as I was developing my program, so you can feel confident about using the recipes and food plan.

Sodium

Most people consume more sodium than their bodies need. The American Heart Association and the American Diabetes Association recommend limiting daily sodium intake to no more than 3,000 milligrams per day. If your doctor suggests you limit your sodium even more, then *you really must read labels.*

Sodium is an essential nutrient and should not be completely eliminated. It helps to regulate blood volume and is needed for normal daily muscle and nerve functions. Most of us, however, have no trouble getting "all we need" and then some.

As with everything else, moderation is my approach. I rarely ever have salt on my list as an added ingredient. But if you're especially sodium-sensitive, make the right choices for you—and save high-sodium foods such as sauerkraut for an occasional treat.

I use lots of spices to enhance flavors, so you won't notice the absence of salt. In the few cases where it is used, salt is vital for the success of the recipe, so please don't omit it.

When I do use an ingredient high in sodium, I try to compensate by using low-sodium products in the remainder of the recipe. Many fat-free products are a little higher in sodium to make up for any loss of flavor that disappeared along with the fat. But when I take advantage of these fat-free, higher-sodium products, I stretch that ingredient within the recipe, lowering the amount of sodium per serving. A good example is my use of fat-free and reduced-sodium canned soups. While the suggested number of servings per can is two, I make sure my final creation serves at least four and sometimes six. So the soup's sodium has been "watered down" from one-third to one-half of the original amount.

Even if you don't have to watch your sodium intake for medical reasons, using moderation is another "healthy exchange" to make on your own journey to good health.

Fat Percentages

We've been told that 30 percent is the magic number—that we should limit fat intake to 30 percent or less of our total calories. It's good advice, and I try to have a weekly average of 15 percent to 25 percent myself. I believe any less than 15 percent is really just another restrictive diet that won't last. And more than 25 percent on a regular basis is too much of a good thing.

When I started listing fat grams along with calories in my recipes, I was tempted to include the percentage of calories from fat. After all, in the vast majority of my recipes, that percentage is well below 30 percent This even includes my pie recipes that allow you a realistic serving instead of many "diet" recipes that tell you a serving is 1/12 of a pie.

Figuring fat grams is easy enough. Each gram of fat equals 9 calories. Multiply fat grams by 9, then divide that number by the total calories to get the percentage of calories from fat.

So why don't I do it? After consulting four registered dietitians for advice, I decided to omit this information. They felt that it's too easy for people to become obsessed by that 30 percent figure, which is after all supposed to be a percentage of total calories over the course of a day or a week. We mustn't feel we can't include a healthy ingredient such as pecans or olives in one recipe just because, on its own, it has more than 30 percent of its calories from fat.

An example of this would be a casserole made with 90 percent lean red meat. Most of us benefit from eating red meat in moderation, as it provides iron and niacin in our diets, and it also makes life more enjoyable for us and those who eat with us. If we *only* look at the percentage of calories from fat in a serving of this one dish, which might be as high as 40 to 45 percent, we might choose not to include this recipe in our weekly food plan.

The dietitians suggested that it's important to consider the total picture when making such decisions. As long as your overall food plan keeps fat calories to 30 percent, it's all right to enjoy an occasional dish that is somewhat higher in fat content. Healthy foods I include in **MODERATION** include 90 percent lean red meat, olives, and nuts. I don't eat these foods every day, and you may not either. But occasionally, in a good recipe, they make all the difference in the world between just getting by (deprivation) and truly enjoying your food.

Remember, the goal is eating in a healthy way so you can enjoy and live well the rest of your life.

Saturated Fats and Cholesterol

You'll see that I don't provide calculations for saturated fats or cholesterol amounts in my recipes. It's for the simple and yet not so simple reason that accurate, up-to-date, brand-specific information can be difficult to obtain from food manufacturers, especially since the way in which they produce food keeps changing rapidly. But once more I've consulted with registered dietitians and other professionals and found that, because I use only a few products that are high in saturated fat, and use them in such limited quantities, my recipes are suitable for patients concerned about controlling or lowering cholesterol. You'll also find that whenever I do use one of these ingredients *in moderation*, everything else in the recipe, and in the meals my family and I enjoy, is low in fat.

Processed Foods

Just what is processed food, anyway? What do I mean by the term "processed food," and why do I use them, when the "purest" recipe developers in Recipe Land consider them "pedestrian" and won't ever use something from a box, container, or can? A letter I received and a passing statement from a stranger made me reflect on what I mean when I refer to processed foods, and helped me reaffirm why I use them in my "common folk" healthy recipes.

If you are like the vast millions who agree with me, then I'm not sharing anything new with you. And if you happen to disagree, that's okay, too. After all, this is America, the Land of the Free. We are blessed to live in a great nation where we can all believe what we want about anything.

A few months go, a woman sent me several articles from various "whole food" publications and wrote that she was wary of processed foods, and wondered why I used them in my recipes. She then scribbled on the bottom of her note, "Just how healthy is Healthy Exchanges?" Then, a few weeks later, during a chance visit at a public food event with a very pleasant woman, I was struck by how we all have our own definitions of what processed foods are. She shared with me, in a somewhat self-righteous manner, that she *never* uses processed foods. She only cooked with fresh fruits and vegetables, she told me. Then later she said that she used canned reduced-fat soups all the time! Was her definition different than mine, I wondered? Soup in a can, whether it's reduced in fat or not, still meets my definition of a processed food.

So I got out a copy of my book *HELP: Healthy Exchanges Lifetime Plan* and reread what I had written back then about processed foods. Nothing in my definition had changed since I wrote that section. I still believe that healthy processed foods, such as canned soups, prepared piecrusts, sugar-free instant puddings, nonfat sour cream, and frozen whipped topping, when used properly, all have a place as ingredients in healthy recipes.

I never use an ingredient that hasn't been approved by either the American Diabetic Association, the American Dietetic Association, or the American Heart Association. Whenever I'm in doubt, I send for their position papers, then ask knowledgeable registered dietitians to explain those papers to me in layman's language. I've been assured by all of them that the sugar- and fat-free products I use in my recipes are indeed safe.

If you don't agree, nothing I can say or write will convince you otherwise. But, if you've been using the healthy processed foods and have been concerned about the almost daily hoopla you hear about yet another product that's going to be the doom of all of us, then just stick with reason. For every product on the grocery shelves, there are those who want you to buy it and there are those who don't, *because they want you to buy their products instead.* So we have to learn to sift the fact from the fiction. Let's take sugar substitutes, for example. In making your own evaluations, you should be skeptical about any information provided by the sugar substitute manufacturers, because they have a vested interest in our buying their products. Likewise, ignore any information provided by the sugar industry, because they have a vested interest in our *not* buying sugar substitutes. Then, if you aren't sure if you can really trust the government or any of its agencies, toss out their data, too. That leaves the three associations I mentioned above. Do you think any of them would say a product is safe if it isn't? Or say a product isn't safe when it is? They have nothing to gain or lose, *other than their integrity,* if they intentionally try to mislead us. That's why I only go to these associations for information concerning healthy processed foods.

I certainly don't recommend that everything we eat should come from a can, box, or jar. I think the best of all possible worlds is to start with the basics: grains such as rice, pasta, or corn. Then, for example, add some raw vegetables and extra-lean meat such as poultry, fish, beef, or pork. Stir in some healthy canned soup or tomato sauce, and you'll end up with something that is not only healthy but tastes so good, everyone from toddlers to great-grandparents will want to eat it!

I've never been in favor of spraying everything we eat with chemicals, and I don't believe that all our foods should come out of packages. But I do think we should use the best available healthy processed foods to make cooking easier and food taste better. I take advantage of the good-tasting low-fat and low-sugar products found in any grocery store. My recipes are created for busy people like me, people who want to eat healthily and economically but who still want the food to satisfy their taste buds. I don't expect anyone to visit out-of-the-way health food stores or find the time to cook beans from scratch—*because I don't!* Most of you can't grow fresh food in the backyard and many of you may not have access to farmers' markets or large supermarkets. I want to help you figure out realistic ways to make healthy eating a reality *wherever you live,* or you will not stick to a healthy lifestyle for long.

So if you've been swayed (by individuals or companies with vested interests or hidden agendas) into thinking that all processed foods are bad for you, you may want to reconsider your position. Or if you've been fooling yourself into believing that you *never* use processed foods but regularly reach for that healthy canned soup, stop playing games with yourself—you are using processed foods in a healthy way. And, if you're like me and use healthy processed foods in *moderation,* don't let anyone make you feel ashamed about including these products in your healthy lifestyle. Only *you* can decide what's best for *you* and your family's needs.

Part of living a healthy lifestyle is making those decisions and then getting on with life. Congratulations on choosing to live a healthy lifestyle, and let's celebrate together by sharing a piece of Healthy Exchanges pie that I've garnished with Cool Whip Lite!

JoAnna's Ten Commandments of Successful Cooking

A very important part of any journey is knowing where you are going and the best way to get there. If you plan and prepare before you start to cook, you should reach mealtime with foods to write home about!

1. **Read the entire recipe from start to finish** and be sure you understand the process involved. Check that you have all the equipment you will need *before* you begin.

2. **Check the ingredient list** and be sure you have *everything* and in the amounts required. Keep cooking sprays handy—while they're not listed as ingredients, I use them all the time (just a quick squirt!).

3. **Set out *all* the ingredients and equipment needed** to prepare the recipe on the counter near you *before* you start. Remember that old saying *A stitch in time saves nine?* It applies in the kitchen, too.

4. **Do as much advance preparation as possible** before actually cooking. Chop, cut, grate, or do whatever is needed to prepare the ingredients and have them ready

before you start to mix. Turn the oven on at least ten minutes before putting food in to bake, to allow the oven to preheat to the proper temperature.

5. **Use a kitchen timer** to tell you when the cooking or baking time is up. Because stove temperatures vary slightly by manufacturer, you may want to set your timer for five minutes less than the suggested time just to prevent overcooking. Check the progress of your dish at that time, then decide if you need the additional minutes or not.

6. **Measure carefully.** Use glass measures for liquids and metal or plastic cups for dry ingredients. My recipes are based on standard measurements. Unless I tell you it's a scant or full cup, measure the cup level.

7. **For best results, follow the recipe instructions exactly.** Feel free to substitute ingredients that *don't tamper* with the basic chemistry of the recipe, but be sure to leave key ingredients alone. For example, you could substitute sugar-free instant chocolate pudding for sugar-free instant butterscotch pudding, but if you used a six-serving package when a four-serving package was listed in the ingredients, or you used instant when cook-and-serve is required, you won't get the right result.

8. **Clean up as you go.** It is much easier to wash a few items at a time than to face a whole counter of dirty dishes later. The same is true for spills on the counter or floor.

9. **Be careful about doubling or halving a recipe.** Though many recipes can be altered successfully to serve more or fewer people, *many cannot.* This is especially true when it comes to spices and liquids. If you try to double a recipe that calls for 1 teaspoon pumpkin pie spice, for example, and you double the spice, you may end up with a too-spicy taste. I usually suggest increasing spices or liquid by 1½ times when doubling a recipe. If it tastes a little bland to you, you can increase the spice to 1¾ times the original amount the next time you prepare the dish. Remember: You can always add more, but you can't take it out after it's stirred in.

The same is true with liquid ingredients. If you wanted to **triple** a recipe like my **Micro Pizza Meatloaf** because you were planning to serve a crowd, you might think you should use three times as much of every ingredient. Don't, or you could end up with Micro Pizza Meatloaf Soup! The original recipe calls for 1¾ cups of chunky tomato sauce, so I'd suggest using 3½ cups when you **triple** the recipe (or 2¾ cups if you **double** it). You'll still have a good-tasting dish that won't run all over the plate.

10. **Write your reactions next to each recipe once you've served it.** Yes, that's right, I'm giving you permission to write in this book. It's yours, after all. Ask yourself: Did everyone like it? Did you have to add another half teaspoon of chili seasoning to please your family, who like to live on the spicier side of the street? You may even want to rate the recipe on a scale of 1☆ to 4☆, depending on what you thought of it. (Four stars would be the top rating—and I hope you'll feel that way about many of my recipes.) Jotting down your comments while they are fresh in your mind will help you personalize the recipe to your own taste the next time you prepare it.

My Best Healthy Exchanges Tips and Tidbits

Measurements, General Cooking Tips, and Basic Ingredients

The word **moderation** best describes **my use of fats, sugar substitutes,** and **sodium** in these recipes. Wherever possible, I've used cooking spray for sautéing and for browning meats and vegetables. I also use reduced-calorie margarine and no-fat mayonnaise and salad dressings. Lean ground turkey *or* ground beef can be used in the recipes. Just be sure whatever you choose is at least *90 percent lean.*

I've also included **small amounts of sugar and brown sugar substitutes as the sweetening agent** in many of the recipes. I don't drink a hundred cans of soda a day or eat enough artificially sweetened foods in a 24-hour time period to be troubled by sugar substitutes. But if this is a concern of yours and you *do not* need to watch your sugar intake, you can always replace the sugar substitutes with processed sugar and the sugar-free products with regular ones.

I created my recipes knowing they would also be used by hypoglycemics, diabetics, and those concerned about triglycerides. If you choose to use sugar instead, be sure to count the additional calories.

A word of caution when cooking with **sugar substitutes**: Use **saccharin**-based sweeteners when **heating or baking**. In recipes that **don't require heat, Aspartame** (known as Nutrasweet) works well in uncooked dishes but leaves an aftertaste in baked products.

I'm often asked why I use an **8-by-8-inch baking dish** in my recipes. It's for portion control. If the recipe says it serves 4, just cut down the center, turn the dish, and cut again. Like magic, there's your serving. Also, if this is the only recipe you are preparing requiring an oven, the square dish fits into a tabletop toaster oven easily and energy can be conserved.

To make life even easier, **whenever a recipe calls for ounce measurements** (other than raw meats) I've included the closest cup equivalent. I need to use my scale daily when creating recipes, so I've measured for you at the same time.

Most of the recipes are for **4 to 6 servings.** If you don't have that many to feed, do what I do: freeze individual portions. Then all you have to do is choose something from the freezer and take it to work for lunch or have your evening meals prepared in advance for the week. In this way, I always have something on hand that is both good to eat and good for me.

Unless a recipe includes hard-boiled eggs, cream cheese, mayonnaise, or a raw vegetable or fruit, **the leftovers should freeze well.** (I've marked recipes that freeze well with the symbol of a **snowflake ❋**.) This includes most of the cream pies. Divide any recipe up into individual servings and freeze for your own "TV" dinners.

Another good idea is **cutting leftover pie into individual pieces and freezing each one separately** in a small Ziploc freezer bag. Then the next time you want to thaw a piece of pie for yourself, you don't have to thaw the whole pie. It's great this way for brown-bag lunches, too. Just pull a piece out of the freezer on your way to work and by lunchtime you will have a wonderful dessert waiting for you.

Unless I specify **"covered" for simmering or baking,** prepare my recipes **uncovered.** Occasionally you will read a recipe that asks you to cover a dish for a time, then to uncover, so read the directions carefully to avoid confusion—and to get the best results.

Low-fat cooking spray is another blessing in a Healthy Exchanges kitchen. It's currently available in three flavors . . .

- **OLIVE-OIL FLAVORED** when cooking Mexican, Italian, or Greek dishes

- **BUTTER FLAVORED** when the hint of butter is desired

- **REGULAR** for everything else.

A quick spray of butter flavored makes air-popped popcorn a low-fat taste treat, or try it as a butter substitute on steaming hot corn on the cob. One light spray of the skillet when browning meat will convince you that you're using "old-fashioned fat," and a quick coating of the casserole dish before you add the ingredients will make serving easier and cleanup quicker.

I use reduced-sodium **canned chicken broth** in place of dry bouillon to lower the sodium content. The intended flavor is still present in the prepared dish. As a reduced-sodium beef broth is not currently available (at least not in DeWitt, Iowa), I use the canned regular beef broth. The sodium content is still lower than regular dry bouillon.

Whenever **cooked rice or pasta** is an ingredient, follow the package directions, but eliminate the salt and/or margarine called for. This helps lower the sodium and fat content. It tastes just fine; trust me on this.

Here's another tip: When **cooking rice or noodles**, why not cook extra "for the pot"? After you use what you need, store leftover rice in a covered container (where it will keep for a couple of days). With noodles like spaghetti or macaroni, first rinse and drain as usual, then measure out what you need. Put the leftovers in a bowl covered with water, then store in the refrigerator, covered, until they're needed. Then, measure out what you need, rinse and drain them, and they're ready to go.

Does your **pita bread** often tear before you can make a sandwich? Here's my tip to make them open easily: cut the bread in half, put the halves in the microwave for about 15 seconds, and they will open up by themselves. *Voilà!*

When **chunky salsa** is listed as an ingredient, I leave the degree of "heat" up to your personal taste. In our house, I'm considered a wimp. I go for the "mild" while Cliff prefers "extra-hot." How do we compromise? I prepare the recipe with mild salsa because he can always add a spoonful or two of the hotter version to his serving, but I can't enjoy the dish if it's too spicy for me.

Milk and Yogurt

Take it from me—nonfat dry milk powder is great! I *do not* use it for drinking, but I *do* use it for cooking. Three good reasons why:

(1) It is very **inexpensive**.

(2) It does not **sour** because you use it only as needed. Store the box in your refrigerator or freezer and it will keep almost forever.

(3) You can easily **add extra calcium** to just about any recipe without added liquid. I consider nonfat dry milk powder one of Mother Nature's modern-day miracles of convenience. But do purchase a good national name brand (I like Carnation), and keep it fresh by proper storage.

In many of my pies and puddings, I use nonfat dry milk powder and water instead of skim milk. Usually I call for ⅔ cup nonfat dry milk powder and 1¼ to 1½ cups water or liquid. This way I can get the nutrients of two cups of milk, but much less liquid, and the end result is much creamier. Also, the recipe sets up quicker, usually in 5 minutes or less. So if someone knocks at your door unexpectedly at mealtime, you can quickly throw a pie together and enjoy it minutes later.

You can make your own "**sour cream**" by combining ¾ cup plain fat-free yogurt with ⅓ cup nonfat dry milk powder. What you did by doing this is fourfold: 1) The dry milk stabilizes the yogurt and keeps the whey from separating. 2) The dry milk slightly helps to cut the tartness of the yogurt. 3) It's still virtually fat-free. 4) The calcium has been increased by 100 percent. Isn't it great how we can make that distant relative of sour cream a first kissin' cousin by adding the nonfat dry milk powder? Or, if you place 1 cup of plain fat-free yogurt in a sieve lined with a coffee filter, and place the sieve over a small bowl and refrigerate for about 6 hours, you will end up with a very good alternative for sour cream. To **stabilize yogurt** when cooking or baking with it, just add 1 teaspoon cornstarch to every ¾ cup yogurt.

If a recipe calls for **evaporated skim milk** and you don't have any in the cupboard, make your own. For every ½ cup evaporated skim milk needed, combine ⅓ cup nonfat dry milk powder and ½ cup water. Use as you would evaporated skim milk.

You can also make your own **sugar-free and fat-free sweetened condensed milk** at home. Combine 1⅓ cups nonfat dry milk powder and ½ cup cold water in a 2-cup glass measure. Cover and microwave on HIGH until mixture is hot but *not* boiling. Stir in ½ cup Sprinkle Sweet or Sugar Twin. Cover and refrigerate at least 4 hours. This mixture will keep for up to two weeks in the refrigerator. Use in just about any recipe that calls for sweetened condensed milk.

For any recipe that calls for **buttermilk**, you might want to try JO's Buttermilk: Blend one cup of water and ⅔ cup dry milk powder (the nutrients of two cups of skim milk). It'll be thicker than this mixed-up milk usually is, because it's doubled. Add 1 teaspoon white vinegar and stir, then let it sit for at least 10 minutes.

One of my subscribers was looking for a way to further restrict salt intake and needed a substitute for **cream of mushroom soup**. For many of my recipes, I use Healthy Request Cream of Mushroom Soup, as it is a reduced-sodium product. The label suggests two servings per can, but I usually incorporate the soup into a recipe serving at least four. By doing this, I've reduced the sodium in the soup by half again.

But if you must restrict your sodium even more, try making my Healthy Exchanges **Creamy Mushroom Sauce.** Place 1½ cups evaporated skim milk and 3 tablespoons flour in a covered jar. Shake well and pour mixture into a medium saucepan sprayed with butter-flavored cooking spray. Add ½ cup canned sliced mushrooms, rinsed and drained. Cook over medium heat, stirring often, until mixture thickens. Add any seasonings of your choice. You can use this sauce in any recipe that calls for one 10¾-ounce can of cream of mushroom soup.

Why did I choose these proportions and ingredients?

- 1½ cups evaporated skim milk is the amount in one can.

- It's equal to three milk choices or exchanges.

- It's the perfect amount of liquid and flour for a medium cream sauce.

- 3 tablespoons flour is equal to one bread/starch choice or exchange.

- Any leftovers will reheat beautifully with a flour-based sauce, but not with a cornstarch base.

- The mushrooms are one vegetable choice or exchange.

- This sauce is virtually fat-free, sugar-free, and sodium-free.

Proteins

I use eggs in moderation. I enjoy the real thing on an average of three to four times a week. So, my recipes are calculated on using whole eggs. However, if you choose to use egg substitute in place of the egg, the finished product will turn out just fine and the fat grams per serving will be even lower than those listed.

If you like the look, taste, and feel of **hard-boiled eggs** in salads but haven't been using them because of the cholesterol in the yolk, I have a couple of alternatives for you. 1) Pour an 8-ounce carton of egg substitute into a medium skillet sprayed with cooking spray. Cover skillet tightly and cook over low heat until substitute is just set, about 10 minutes. Remove from heat and let set, still covered, for 10 minutes more. Uncover and cool completely. Chop set mixture. This will make about 1 cup of chopped egg. 2) Even easier is to hard-boil "real eggs," toss the yolk away, and chop the white. Either way, you don't deprive yourself of the pleasure of egg in your salad.

In most recipes calling for **egg substitutes**, you can use 2 egg whites in place of the equivalent of 1 egg substitute. Just break the eggs open and toss the yolks away. I can hear some of you already saying, "But that's wasteful!" Well, take a look at the price on the egg substitute package (which usually has the equivalent of 4 eggs in it), then look at the price of a dozen eggs, from which you'd get the equivalent of 6 egg substitutes. Now, what's wasteful about that?

Whenever I include **cooked chicken** in a recipe, I use roasted white meat without skin. Whenever I include **roast beef or pork** in a recipe, I use the loin cuts because they are much leaner. However, most of the time, I do my roasting of all these meats at the local deli. I just ask for a chunk of their lean roasted meat, 6 or 8 ounces, and ask them not to slice it. When I get home, I cube or dice the meat and am ready to use it in my recipe. The reason I do this is three-fold: 1) I'm getting just the amount I need without leftovers; 2) I don't have the expense of heating the oven; and 3) I'm not throwing away the bone, gristle, and fat I'd be cutting off the meat. Overall, it is probably cheaper to "roast" it the way I do.

Did you know that you can make an acceptable meatloaf without using egg for the binding? Just replace every egg with ¼ cup of liquid. You could use beef broth, tomato sauce, even applesauce, to name just a few. For a meatloaf to serve 6, I always use 1 pound of extra-lean ground beef or turkey, 6 tablespoons of dried fine bread crumbs, and ¼ cup of the liquid, plus anything else healthy that strikes my fancy at the time. I mix well and place the mixture in an 8-by-8-inch baking dish or 9-by-5-inch loaf pan sprayed with cooking spray. Bake uncovered at 350 degrees for 35 to 50 minutes (depending on the added ingredients). You will never miss the egg.

Any time you are **browning ground meat** for a casserole and want to get rid of almost all the excess fat, just place the uncooked meat loosely in a plastic colander. Set the colander in a glass pie plate. Place in microwave and cook on HIGH for 3 to 6 minutes (depending on the amount being browned), stirring often. Use as you would for any casserole. You can also chop up onions and brown them with the meat if you want.

Fruits and Vegetables

If you want to enjoy a **"fruit shake"** with some pizazz, just combine soda water and unsweetened fruit juice in a blender. Add crushed ice. Blend on HIGH until thick. Refreshment without guilt.

You'll see that many recipes use ordinary **canned vegetables.** They're much cheaper than reduced-sodium versions, and once you rinse and drain them, the sodium is reduced anyway. I believe in saving money wherever possible so we can afford the best fat-free and sugar-free products as they come onto the market.

All three kinds of **vegetables—fresh, frozen, and canned—** have their place in a healthy diet. My husband, Cliff, hates the taste of frozen or fresh green beans, thinks the texture is all wrong, so I use canned green beans instead. In this case, canned vegetables have their proper place when I'm feeding my husband. If someone in your family has a similar concern, it's important to respond to it so everyone can be happy and enjoy the meal.

When I use **fruits or vegetables** like apples, cucumbers, and zucchini, I wash them really well and **leave the skin on.** It provides added color, fiber, and attractiveness to any dish. And, because I use processed flour in my cooking, I like to increase the fiber in my diet by eating my fruits and vegetables in their closest-to-natural state.

To help keep **fresh fruits and veggies fresh**, just give them a quick "shower" with lemon juice. The easiest way to do this is to pour purchased lemon juice into a kitchen spray bottle and store in the refrigerator. Then, every time you use fresh fruits or vegetables in a salad or dessert, simply give them a quick spray with your "lemon spritzer." You just might be amazed by how this little trick keeps your produce from turning brown so fast.

The next time you warm canned vegetables such as carrots or green beans, drain and heat the vegetables in ¼ cup beef or chicken broth. It gives a nice variation to an old standby. Here's a simple **white sauce** for vegetables and casseroles without using added fat that can be made by spraying a medium saucepan with butter-flavored cooking spray. Place 1½ cups evaporated skim milk and 3 tablespoons flour in a covered jar. Shake well. Pour into sprayed saucepan and cook over medium heat until thick, stirring constantly. Add salt and pepper to taste. You can also add ½ cup canned drained mushrooms and/or 3 ounces (¾ cup) shredded reduced-fat cheese. Continue cooking until cheese melts.

Zip up canned or frozen green beans with **chunky salsa**: ½ cup to 2 cups beans. Heat thoroughly. Chunky salsa also makes a wonderful dressing on lettuce salads. It only counts as a vegetable, so enjoy.

Another wonderful **South of the Border** dressing can be stirred up by using ½ cup of chunky salsa and ¼ cup fat-free Ranch dressing. Cover and store in your refrigerator. Use as a dressing for salads or as a topping for baked potatoes.

For **gravy** with all the "old time" flavor but without the extra fat, try this almost effortless way to prepare it. (It's almost as easy as opening up a store-bought jar.) Pour the juice off your roasted meat, then set the roast aside to "rest" for about 20 minutes. Place the juice in an uncovered cake pan or other large flat pan (we want the large air surface to speed up the cooling process) and put in the freezer until the fat congeals on top and you can skim it off. Or, if you prefer, use a skimming pitcher purchased at your kitchen gadget store. Either way, measure about 1½ cups skimmed broth and pour into a medium saucepan. Cook over medium heat until heated through, about 5 minutes. In a covered jar, combine ½ cup water or cooled potato broth with 3 tablespoons flour. Shake well. Pour flour mixture into warmed juice. Combine well using a wire whisk. Continue cooking until gravy thickens, about 5 minutes. Season with salt and pepper to taste.

Why did I use flour instead of cornstarch? Because any left-overs will reheat nicely with the flour base and would not with a cornstarch base. Also, 3 tablespoons of flour works out to 1 Bread/Starch exchange. This virtually fat-free gravy makes about 2 cups, so you could spoon about ½ cup gravy on your low-fat mashed potatoes and only have to count your gravy as ¼ Bread/Starch exchange.

Desserts

Thaw **lite whipped topping** in the refrigerator overnight. Never try to force the thawing by stirring or using a microwave to soften. Stirring it will remove the air from the topping that gives it the lightness and texture we want, and there's not enough fat in it to survive being heated.

How can I **frost an entire pie with just ½ cup of whipped topping?** First, don't use an inexpensive brand. I use Cool Whip Lite or La Creme Lite. Make sure the topping is fully thawed. Always spread from the center to the sides using a rubber spatula. This way, ½ cup topping will literally cover an entire pie. Remember, the operative word is *frost*, not pile the entire container on top of the pie!

For a special treat that tastes anything but "diet," try placing **spreadable fruit** in a container and microwave for about 15 seconds. Then pour the melted fruit spread over a serving of nonfat ice cream or frozen yogurt. One tablespoon of spreadable fruit is equal to 1 fruit serving. Some combinations to get you started are apricot over chocolate ice cream, strawberry over strawberry ice cream, or any flavor over vanilla.

Another way I use spreadable fruit is to make a delicious **topping for a cheesecake or angel food cake**. I take ½ cup of fruit and ½ cup Cool Whip Lite and blend the two together with a teaspoon of coconut extract.

Here's a really **good topping** for the fall of the year. Place 1½ cups unsweetened applesauce in a medium saucepan or 4-cup glass measure. Stir in 2 tablespoons raisins, 1 teaspoon apple pie spice, and 2 tablespoons Cary's Sugar Free Maple Syrup. Cook over medium heat on stove or process on HIGH in microwave until warm. Then spoon about ½ cup warm mixture over pancakes, French toast, or fat-free and sugar-free vanilla ice cream. It's as close as you will get to guilt-free apple pie!

A quick yet tasty way to prepare **strawberries for shortcake** is to place about ¾ cup sliced strawberries, 2 tablespoons Diet Mountain Dew, and sugar substitute to equal ¼ cup sugar in a blender container. Process on BLEND until mixture is smooth. Pour mixture into bowl. Add 1¼ cups sliced strawberries and mix well. Cover and refrigerate until ready to serve with shortcake.

The next time you are making treats for the family, try using **unsweetened applesauce** for some or all of the required oil in the recipe. For instance, if the recipe calls for ½ cup cooking oil, use up to the ½ cup in applesauce. It works and most people will not even notice the difference. It's great in purchased cake mixes, but so far I haven't been able to figure out a way to deep-fat fry with it!

Another trick I often use is to include tiny amounts of "real people" food, such as coconut, but extend the flavor by using extracts. Try it—you will be surprised by how little of the real thing you can use and still feel you are not being deprived.

If you are preparing a pie filling that has ample moisture, just line **graham crackers** in the bottom of a 9-by-9-inch cake pan. Pour the filling over the top of the crackers. Cover and refrigerate until the moisture has enough time to soften the crackers. Overnight is best. This eliminates the added **fats and sugars of a piecrust.**

When **stirring fat-free cream cheese to soften it**, use only a sturdy spoon, never an electric mixer. The speed of a mixer can cause the cream cheese to lose its texture and become watery.

Did you know you can make your own **fruit-flavored yogurt?** Mix 1 tablespoon of any flavor of spreadable fruit spread with ¾ cup plain yogurt. It's every bit as tasty and much cheaper. You can also make your own **lemon yogurt** by combining 3 cups plain fat-free yogurt with 1 tub Crystal Light lemonade powder. Mix well, cover, and store in refrigerator. I think you will be pleasantly surprised by the ease, cost, and flavor of this "made from scratch" calcium-rich treat. P.S.: You can make any flavor you like by using any of the Crystal Light mixes—Cranberry? Iced Tea? You decide.

Sugar-free puddings and gelatins are important to many of my recipes, but if you prefer to avoid sugar substitutes, you could still prepare the recipes with regular puddings or gelatins. The calories would be higher, but you would still be cooking low-fat.

When a recipe calls for **chopped nuts** (and you only have whole ones), who wants to dirty the food processor just for a couple of tablespoonsful? You could try to chop them using your cutting board, but be prepared for bits and pieces to fly all over the kitchen. I use "Grandma's food processor." I take the biggest nuts I can find, put them in a small glass bowl, and chop them into chunks just the right size using a metal biscuit cutter.

If you have a **leftover muffin** and are looking for something a little different for breakfast, you can make **a "breakfast sundae."** Crumble the muffin into a cereal bowl. Sprinkle a serving of fresh fruit over it and top with a couple of tablespoons of nonfat plain yogurt sweetened with sugar substitute and your choice of extract. The thought of it just might make you jump out of bed with a smile on your face. (Speaking of muffins, did you know that if you fill the unused muffin wells with water when baking muffins, you help ensure more even baking and protect the muffin pan at the same time?) Another muffin hint: Lightly spray the inside of paper baking cups with butter-flavored cooking spray before spooning the muffin batter into them. Then you won't end up with paper clinging to your fresh-baked muffins.

The secret of making **good meringues** without sugar is to use 1 tablespoon of Sprinkle Sweet or Sugar Twin for every egg white, and a small amount of extract. Use ½ to 1 teaspoon for the batch. Almond, vanilla, and coconut are all good choices. Use the same amount of cream of tartar you usually do. Bake the meringue in the same old way. Don't think you can't have meringue pies because you can't eat sugar. You can, if you do it my way. (Remember that egg whites whip up best at room temperature.)

Homemade or Store-Bought?

I've been asked which is better for you: homemade from scratch, or purchased foods. My answer is *both!* Each has a place in a healthy lifestyle, and what that place is has everything to do with you.

Take **piecrusts**, for instance. If you love spending your spare time in the kitchen preparing foods, and you're using low-fat, low-sugar, and reasonably low sodium ingredients, go for it! But if, like so many people, your time is limited and you've learned to read labels, you could be better off using purchased foods.

I know that when I prepare a pie (and I experiment with a couple of pies each week, because this is Cliff's favorite dessert), I use a purchased crust. Why? Mainly because I can't make a good-tasting piecrust that is lower in fat than the brands I use. Also, purchased piecrusts fit my rule of "If it takes longer to fix than to eat, forget it!"

I've checked the nutrient information for the purchased piecrusts against recipes for traditional and "diet" piecrusts, using my computer software program. The purchased crust calculated lower in both fat and calories! I have tried some low-fat and low-sugar recipes, but they just didn't spark my taste buds, or were so complicated you needed an engineering degree just to get the crust in the pie plate.

I'm very happy with the purchased piecrusts in my recipes, because the finished product rarely, if ever, has more than 30 percent of total calories coming from fats. I also believe that we have to prepare foods our families and friends will eat with us on a regular basis and not feel deprived, or we've wasted time, energy, and money.

I could use a purchased "lite" **pie filling**, but instead I make my own. Here I can save both fat and sugar, and still make the filling almost as fast as opening a can. The bottom line: Know what you have to spend when it comes to both time and fat/sugar calories, then make the best decision you can for you and your family. And don't go without an occasional piece of pie because you think it isn't *necessary*. A delicious pie prepared in a healthy way is one of the simple pleasures of life. It's a little thing, but it can make all the difference between just getting by with the bare minimum and living a full and healthy lifestyle.

Many people have experimented with my tip about **substituting applesauce and artificial sweetener for butter and sugar**, but what if you aren't satisfied with the result? One woman wrote to me about a recipe for her grandmother's cookies that called for 1 cup of butter and 1½ cups of sugar. Well, any recipe that depends on as much butter and sugar as this one does is generally not a good candidate for "healthy exchanges." The original recipe needed a large quantity of fat to produce a crisp cookie just like Grandma made.

Unsweetened applesauce can be used to substitute for vegetable oil with various degrees of success, but not to replace butter, lard, or margarine. If your recipe calls for ½ cup oil or less, and it's a quick bread, muffin, or bar cookie, it should work to replace the oil with applesauce. If the recipe calls for more than ½ cup oil, then experiment with half oil, half applesauce. You've still made the recipe healthier, even if you haven't removed all the oil from it.

Another rule for healthy substitution: Up to ½ cup sugar or less can be replaced by *an artificial sweetener that can withstand the heat of baking*, like Sugar Twin or Sprinkle Sweet. If it requires more than ½ cup sugar, cut the amount needed by 75 percent and use ½ cup sugar substitute and sugar for the rest. Other options: Reduce the butter and sugar by 25 percent and see if the finished product still satisfies you in taste and appearance. Or, make the cookies just like Grandma did, realizing they are part of your family's holiday tradition. Enjoy a moderate serving of a couple of cookies once or twice during the season, and just forget about them the rest of the year.

I'm sure you'll add to this list of cooking tips as you begin preparing Healthy Exchanges recipes and discover how easy it can be to adapt your own favorite recipes using these ideas and your own common sense.

A Peek into My Pantry and My Favorite Brands

Everyone asks me what foods I keep on hand and what brands I use. There are lots of good products on the grocery shelves today—many more than we dreamed about even a year or two ago. And I can't wait to see what's out there twelve months from now. The following are my staples and, where appropriate, my favorites *at this time*. I feel these products are healthier, tastier, easy to get—and deliver the most flavor for the least amount of fat, sugar, or calories. If you find others you like as well *or better,* please use them. This is only a guide to make your grocery shopping and cooking easier.

Fat-free plain yogurt (*Yoplait or Dannon*)
Nonfat dry skim milk powder (*Carnation*)
Evaporated skim milk (*Carnation*)
Skim milk
Fat-free cottage cheese
Fat-free cream cheese (*Philadelphia*)
Fat-free mayonnaise (*Kraft*)
Fat-free salad dressings (*Kraft*)
Fat-free sour cream (*Land O Lakes*)
Reduced-calorie margarine (*Weight Watchers, Promise, or Smart Beat*)
Cooking spray
    Olive-oil flavored and regular (*Pam*)
    Butter flavored for sautéing (*Weight Watchers*)

Butter flavored for spritzing *after* cooking (*I Can't Believe It's Not Butter!*)

Vegetable oil (*Puritan Canola Oil*)

Reduced-calorie whipped topping (*Cool Whip Lite or Cool Whip Free*)

Sugar substitute
  if no heating is involved (*Equal*)
  if heating is required
      white (*Sugar Twin or Sprinkle Sweet*)
      brown (*Brown Sugar Twin*)

Sugar-free gelatin and pudding mixes (*JELL-O*)

Baking mix (*Bisquick Reduced Fat*)

Pancake mix (*Aunt Jemima Reduced-Calorie*)

Reduced-calorie pancake syrup (*Cary's Sugar Free*)

Parmesan cheese (*Kraft fat-free*)

Reduced-fat cheese (*Kraft ⅓ Less Fat*)

Shredded frozen potatoes (*Mr. Dell's*)

Spreadable fruit spread (*Smucker's, Welch's, or Knott's Berry Farm*)

Peanut butter (*Peter Pan reduced-fat, Jif reduced-fat, or Skippy reduced-fat*)

Chicken broth (*Healthy Request*)

Beef broth (*Swanson*)

Tomato sauce (*Hunt's—plain, Italian, or chili*)

Canned soups (*Healthy Request*)

Tomato juice (*Campbell's Reduced-Sodium*)

Ketchup (*Heinz Light Harvest or Healthy Choice*)

Purchased piecrust
  unbaked (*Pillsbury—from dairy case*)
  graham cracker, butter-flavored, or chocolate-flavored (*Keebler*)

Crescent rolls (*Pillsbury Reduced Fat*)

Pastrami and corned beef (*Carl Buddig Lean*)

Luncheon meats (*Healthy Choice or Oscar Mayer*)

Ham (*Dubuque 97% fat-free and reduced-sodium or Healthy Choice*)

Frankfurters and Kielbasa sausage (*Healthy Choice*)

Canned white chicken, packed in water (*Swanson*)

Canned tuna, packed in water (*Chicken of the Sea*)

90–95 percent lean ground turkey and beef
Soda crackers (*Nabisco Fat-Free*)
Reduced-calorie bread—40 calories per slice or less
Hamburger buns—80 calories each (*Less*)
Rice—instant, regular, brown, and wild
Instant potato flakes (*Betty Crocker Potato Buds*)
Noodles, spaghetti, and macaroni
Salsa (*Chi Chi's Mild Chunky*)
Pickle relish—dill, sweet, and hot dog
Mustard—Dijon, prepared, and spicy
Unsweetened apple juice
Unsweetened applesauce
Fruit—fresh, frozen (no sugar added), or canned in juice
Vegetables—fresh, frozen, or canned
Spices—JO's Spices
Lemon and lime juice (in small plastic fruit-shaped bottles
    found in produce section)
Instant fruit beverage mixes (*Crystal Light*)
Dry dairy beverage mixes (*Nestlé's Quik and Swiss Miss*)
"Ice Cream"—*Well's Blue Bunny sugar- and fat-free*

The items on my shopping list are everyday foods found in just about any grocery store in America. But all are as low in fat, sugar, calories, and sodium as I can find—and still taste good! I can make any recipe in my cookbooks and newsletters as long as I have my cupboards and refrigerator stocked with these items. Whenever I use the last of any one item, I just make sure I pick up another supply the next time I'm at the store.

If your grocer does not stock these items, why not ask if they can be ordered on a trial basis? If the store agrees to do so, be sure to tell your friends to stop by, so that sales are good enough to warrant restocking the new products. Competition for shelf space is fierce, so only products that sell well stay around.

How to Read a Healthy Exchanges Recipe

The Healthy Exchanges Nutritional Analysis

Before using these recipes, you may wish to consult your physician or health-care provider to be sure they are appropriate for you. The information in this book is not intended to take the place of any medical advice. It reflects my experiences, studies, research, and opinions regarding healthy eating.

Each recipe includes nutritional information calculated in three ways:

Healthy Exchanges Weight Loss Choices™ or Exchanges
Calories, fiber, and fat grams
Diabetic exchanges

In every Healthy Exchanges recipe, the diabetic exchanges have been calculated by a registered dietitian. All the other calculations were done by computer, using the Food Processor II software. When the ingredient listing gives more than one choice, the first ingredient listed is the one used in the recipe analysis. Due to inevitable variations in the ingredients you choose to use, the nutritional values should be considered approximate.

The annotation "(limited)" following Protein counts in some recipes indicates that consumption of whole eggs should be limited to four per week.

Please note the following symbols:

☆ This star means read the recipe's directions carefully for special instructions about **division** of ingredients.

✳ This symbol indicates **FREEZES WELL.**

Soups

Garlic Soup

Ever follow your nose to a little, out-of-the-way restaurant just because it smelled so good? You may find your family peeking into your kitchen while you're cooking this soup; it's that fragrant and rich tasting!   ☻   Serves 4

½ cup finely chopped onion
4 cups (two 16-ounce cans) Healthy Request Chicken Broth
6 cloves garlic, minced, or 2 teaspoons dried minced garlic
¼ teaspoon black pepper
2 eggs, beaten, or equivalent in egg substitute
½ cup (¾ ounce) purchased herb-seasoned dried bread cubes
¼ cup chopped fresh parsley or 1 tablespoon dried parsley flakes

In a large saucepan sprayed with butter-flavored cooking spray, sauté onion for 5 minutes or until tender. Add chicken broth, garlic, and black pepper. Bring mixture to a boil. Lower heat, cover, and simmer for 20 minutes. Slowly pour eggs into hot soup in a thin stream, stirring very gently until eggs set. For each serving, place about 2 tablespoons bread cubes into a soup bowl, spoon about 1 cup of soup over top, and garnish with 1 tablespoon parsley. Serve at once.

HINT: Pepperidge Farm bread cubes work great.

Each serving equals:

HE: ½ Protein (limited) • ¼ Vegetable • ¼ Bread •
16 Optional Calories

---

95 Calories • 3 gm Fat • 8 gm Protein •
9 gm Carbohydrate • 582 mg Sodium •
37 mg Calcium • 1 gm Fiber

DIABETIC: ½ Meat • ½ Starch

Egg and Spinach Soup

This delicate but delectable dish couldn't be simpler to prepare, and its unique combination of flavors will win over your taste buds in just a spoonful! This is one case where you need fresh spinach—the frozen kind just won't do.   ☕   Serves 4 (1 full cup)

4 cups (two 16-ounce cans) Healthy Request Chicken Broth
¼ teaspoon lemon pepper
1 cup chopped fresh spinach leaves, stems discarded
1 egg, slightly beaten, or equivalent in egg substitute

In a medium saucepan, combine chicken broth and lemon pepper. Bring mixture to a boil. Stir in spinach leaves. Slowly pour egg into hot soup in a thin stream, stirring very gently until egg is set. Serve at once.

Each serving equals:

HE: ½ Vegetable • ¼ Protein (limited) •
16 Optional Calories

---

33 Calories • 1 gm Fat • 5 gm Protein •
1 gm Carbohydrate • 496 mg Sodium •
6 mg Calcium • 0 gm Fiber

DIABETIC: 1 Free Food

Creamy Vegetable Chowder

Here's a soup so thick and luscious, everyone will be sure you've been standing over a hot stove for *hours!* It's so full of creamy goodness, no one will notice that it also delivers a nice big serving of healthy veggies too. ❍ Serves 4 (1¼ cups)

> 2 cups (one 16-ounce can) Healthy Request Chicken Broth
> 1 cup water
> 1 cup (5 ounces) diced raw potatoes
> ½ cup frozen peas
> ½ cup frozen corn
> ½ cup chopped onion
> ¾ cup finely diced celery
> ¾ cup shredded carrots
> 1 cup frozen cut green beans
> 1½ cups (one 12-fluid-ounce can) Carnation Evaporated Skim Milk
> 3 tablespoons all-purpose flour
> ½ teaspoon lemon pepper
> 2 teaspoons dried parsley flakes

In a large saucepan, combine chicken broth, water, potatoes, peas, corn, onion, celery, carrots, and green beans. Bring mixture to a boil. Lower heat and simmer for 15 to 20 minutes or until vegetables are tender. In a covered jar, combine evaporated skim milk and flour. Shake well to blend. Add milk mixture to vegetable mixture. Mix well to combine. Stir in lemon pepper. Continue simmering until mixture thickens, stirring often. When serving, sprinkle ½ teaspoon parsley flakes over top of each bowl.

Each serving equals:

HE: 1½ Vegetable • 1 Bread • ¾ Skim Milk •
8 Optional Calories

180 Calories • 0 gm Fat • 12 gm Protein •
33 gm Carbohydrate • 387 mg Sodium •
318 mg Calcium • 4 gm Fiber

DIABETIC: 1 Vegetable • 1 Starch • 1 Skim Milk

Allie's Kozy Minestrone Soup

Minestrone is such a great old-fashioned kind of soup, one where you toss in an abundance of different veggies you have on hand and produce an unforgettable meal-in-a-bowl! Elbow macaroni is a good choice, but if you've got some rotini in the cupboard, that would be welcome instead.   ☻   Serves 6 (1½ cups)

> 4 cups water☆
> 1 cup chopped onion
> 1 cup chopped celery
> 1 clove garlic, minced, or ½ teaspoon dried minced garlic
> 3½ cups (two 15-ounce cans) Hunt's Recipe Ready Tomatoes
> 1 cup (one 8-ounce can) Hunt's Tomato Sauce
> 6 ounces (one 8-ounce can) red kidney beans, rinsed and drained
> 2 cups chopped broccoli
> 1½ cups diced carrots
> ¼ cup chopped parsley or
>   1 tablespoon dried parsley flakes
> 1½ teaspoons Italian seasoning
> ½ teaspoon black pepper
> ¾ cup (1½ ounces) uncooked macaroni

In a large saucepan, bring ½ cup water to a boil. Add onion, celery, and garlic. Mix well to combine. Cook for 5 minutes, stirring often. Stir in undrained tomatoes, tomato sauce, kidney beans, remaining 3½ cups water, broccoli, carrots, parsley, Italian seasoning, and black pepper. Lower heat and simmer for 20 minutes. Stir in uncooked macaroni. Continue simmering for 15 minutes or until macaroni is tender.

Each serving equals:

HE: 3⅓ Vegetable • ½ Protein • ⅓ Bread

177 Calories • 1 gm Fat • 9 gm Protein •
33 gm Carbohydrate • 514 mg Sodium •
48 mg Calcium • 8 gm Fiber

DIABETIC: 3 Vegetable • 1 Starch • ½ Meat

Creamy Corn Chowder

Ease of preparation makes sense for anyone with a busy schedule, but it's especially important for everyone coping with achy joints. Armed with an electric can opener and your trusty spice rack, you can stir up this appetizing soup in no time at all!

⊙ Serves 2 (1 full cup)

1 cup (one 8-ounce can) cream-style corn

1 cup (one 8-ounce can) whole-kernel corn, undrained

1 teaspoon dried onion flakes

⅓ cup Carnation Nonfat Dry Milk Powder

¼ cup water

½ teaspoon dried parsley flakes

¼ teaspoon black pepper

In a small saucepan, combine cream-style corn, undrained whole-kernel corn, onion flakes, dry milk powder, water, parsley flakes, and black pepper. Cook over medium heat until mixture is heated through, stirring often.

HINT: Also good with ½ cup (3 ounces) diced extra-lean ham added.

Each serving equals:

HE: 2 Bread • ½ Skim Milk

---

200 Calories • 0 gm Fat • 8 gm Protein •
42 gm Carbohydrate • 431 mg Sodium •
148 mg Calcium • 4 gm Fiber

DIABETIC: 2 Starch • ½ Skim Milk

Corn and Crab Chowder

It used to be that seafood chowders were enjoyed only on special occasions and vacations to the seaside, but now that tasty canned crabmeat is available just about everywhere, this hearty but sophisticated soup is a great choice for an anytime treat! If the mixture thickens up too much, you can add a few drops of water.

Serves 2

1 (4½-ounce drained weight) can crabmeat, rinsed and drained
2 cups skim milk
1 cup (one 8-ounce can) cream-style corn
1 tablespoon dried onion flakes
¼ teaspoon dried minced garlic
⅓ cup (¾ ounce) instant potato flakes

In a medium saucepan, combine crabmeat, skim milk, corn, onion flakes, and garlic. Cook over medium heat until mixture is hot, but not boiling, stirring often. Stir in instant potato flakes. Lower heat and simmer for 5 minutes, or until mixture thickens and is heated through, stirring often.

HINT: Canned tuna or chicken may be substituted for crabmeat.

Each serving equals:

HE: 2 Protein • 1½ Bread • 1 Skim Milk

290 Calories • 2 gm Fat • 26 gm Protein •
42 gm Carbohydrate • 940 mg Sodium •
333 mg Calcium • 2 gm Fiber

DIABETIC: 2 Meat • 2 Starch • 1 Skim Milk

Turkey Chowder

Wouldn't this be a tasty way to greet the New Year, using up some leftover holiday turkey in a mouth-watering soup so luscious you may just keep all those resolutions? If one of your promises to yourself is to eat healthy from now on, why not start with this?

☻ Serves 6 (1½ cups)

> 2 cups (10 ounces) sliced raw potatoes
>
> 1½ cups sliced onion
>
> 2 cups (one 16-ounce can) Healthy Request Chicken Broth
>
> ½ teaspoon poultry seasoning
>
> ⅛ teaspoon black pepper
>
> 3 cups (two 12-fluid-ounce cans) Carnation Evaporated Skim Milk
>
> 2 cups (one 16-ounce can) cream-style corn
>
> 2 full cups (12 ounces) diced cooked turkey breast

In a large saucepan, combine potatoes, onion, chicken broth, poultry seasoning, and black pepper. Cook over medium heat until potatoes are tender. Add evaporated skim milk, corn, and turkey. Mix well to combine. Lower heat and simmer for 15 minutes, stirring occasionally.

HINT: If you don't have leftovers, purchase a chunk of cooked turkey breast from your local deli.

Each serving equals:

HE: 2 Protein • 1 Bread • 1 Skim Milk • ½ Vegetable • 5 Optional Calories

---

302 Calories • 2 gm Fat • 31 gm Protein • 40 gm Carbohydrate • 595 mg Sodium • 393 mg Calcium • 2 gm Fiber

---

DIABETIC: 2 Meat • 1½ Starch • 1 Skim Milk

Turkey-Vegetable Soup

There's something so old-timey and cozy about a long-cooking vegetable soup, especially when it's thick with chunks of turkey that make it extra-hearty! On those days when there isn't time for *anything*, you can still nourish yourself and your family well.

Serves 6 (1 full cup)

> 2 full cups (12 ounces) diced cooked turkey breast
> 4 cups (two 16-ounce cans) Healthy Request Chicken Broth
> 1½ cups water
> ½ teaspoon lemon pepper
> 1 teaspoon dried parsley flakes
> ¾ cup chopped onion
> 1½ cups finely diced celery
> 1¾ cups finely chopped carrots
> ½ cup (one 2.5-ounce jar) sliced mushrooms, drained

In a slow cooker container, combine turkey, chicken broth, water, lemon pepper, and parsley flakes. Stir in onion, celery, carrots, and mushrooms. Cover and cook on LOW for 8 hours. Mix well before serving.

HINT: If you don't have leftovers, purchase a chunk of cooked turkey breast from your local deli.

Each serving equals:

HE: 2 Protein • 1⅓ Vegetable • 11 Optional Calories

130 Calories • 2 gm Fat • 21 gm Protein •
7 gm Carbohydrate • 456 mg Sodium •
36 mg Calcium • 2 gm Fiber

DIABETIC: 2 Meat • 1 Vegetable

Pennsylvania Dutch Chicken Corn Soup

If you visit just about any of the family-style restaurants in rural Pennsylvania, you're bound to find homemade chicken corn soup on the bill of fare! This one takes very little work on your part, but it tastes so richly old-fashioned, everyone will be warmed all the way through. ☻ Serves 4 (1¼ cups)

> 4 cups (two 16-ounce cans) Healthy Request Chicken Broth
> ½ cup chopped onion
> ½ cup finely chopped celery
> 8 ounces skinned and boned uncooked chicken breast, cut into 12 pieces
> ¼ teaspoon black pepper
> ¼ teaspoon dried basil
> 1 cup frozen whole-kernel corn
> 1 scant cup (1½ ounces) uncooked fine noodles
> 1 hard-boiled egg, chopped
> 1 tablespoon chopped fresh parsley or 1 teaspoon dried parsley flakes

In a large saucepan, combine chicken broth, onion, celery, and chicken pieces. Cook over medium heat until chicken is tender, about 10 minutes. Stir in black pepper and basil. Add corn and uncooked noodles. Mix well to combine. Bring mixture to a boil. Lower heat, cover, and simmer for 10 minutes, or until noodles and vegetables are tender, stirring occasionally. Remove from heat. Stir in egg and parsley. Serve at once.

HINT: If you want the look and feel of egg without the cholesterol, toss out the yolk and dice the white.

Each serving equals:

HE: 1¾ Protein (¼ limited) • 1 Bread • ½ Vegetable •
16 Optional Calories

199 Calories • 3 gm Fat • 21 gm Protein •
22 gm Carbohydrate • 551 mg Sodium •
32 mg Calcium • 2 gm Fiber

DIABETIC: 2 Meat • 1 Starch

Celery Chicken Soup

Here's a wonderfully yummy chicken noodle soup made even more delicious by the addition of lots of celery. If you're trying to make sure you include more vegetables in your daily menu, this dish—with *two* servings in just one bowl—is a real winner!

◐ Serves 4 (1½ cups)

> 4 cups (two 16-ounce cans) Healthy Request Chicken Broth
> 1 cup chopped onion
> 3 cups diced celery
> 1 cup (5 ounces) diced cooked chicken breast
> 2 tablespoons dried parsley flakes
> ⅛ teaspoon black pepper
> 1¾ cups (3 ounces) uncooked medium noodles

In a large saucepan, combine chicken broth, onion, celery, chicken, parsley flakes, and black pepper. Bring mixture to a boil. Lower heat and simmer for 15 minutes. Add noodles. Mix well to combine. Cover and continue simmering for 10 minutes or until vegetables and noodles are tender, stirring occasionally.

HINT: If you don't have leftovers, purchase a chunk of cooked chicken breast from your local deli.

Each serving equals:

HE: 2 Vegetable • 1¼ Protein • 1 Bread •
16 Optional Calories

---

123 Calories • 2 gm Fat • 14 gm Protein •
12 gm Carbohydrate • 337 mg Sodium •
66 mg Calcium • 3 gm Fiber

DIABETIC: 1 Vegetable • 1 Meat • 1 Starch

Spinach Chicken Rice Soup

Spinach is such a good-for-you vegetable, I'm always looking for ways to include it in my recipes. This soup is a perfect choice for a weekend supper: the ingredients are simple and usually right at hand, and when these tasty flavors simmer up together, you'll be delightfully satisfied with your quick-fix meal.

☻ Serves 4 (1½ cups)

4 cups (two 16-ounce cans) Healthy Request Chicken Broth
1½ cups hot cooked rice
1 (10-ounce) package frozen chopped spinach, thawed and
*   thoroughly drained*
1 cup (5 ounces) diced cooked chicken breast
¼ teaspoon black pepper
¼ cup (¾ ounce) grated Kraft fat-free Parmesan cheese

In a large saucepan, combine chicken broth, rice, spinach, chicken, and black pepper. Bring mixture to a boil. Lower heat and simmer for 15 minutes. When serving, garnish each bowl with 1 tablespoon Parmesan cheese.

HINTS: 1. 1 cup of uncooked rice usually cooks to about 1½ cups.
2. Thaw spinach by placing in a colander and rinsing under hot water for one minute.
3. If you don't have leftovers, purchase a chunk of cooked chicken breast from your local deli.

Each serving equals:

HE: 1 Protein • ¾ Bread • ½ Vegetable •
16 Optional Calories

170 Calories • 2 gm Fat • 18 gm Protein •
20 gm Carbohydrate • 640 mg Sodium •
89 mg Calcium • 3 gm Fiber

DIABETIC: 2 Meat • 1 Starch • 1 Vegetable

Altrurian Vegetable Beef Soup

Healthy cooking is sometimes so wonderfully easy—you start with a few good-tasting ingredients, add a touch of spice and some fat-free magic, and simply simmer! The flavorful and filling result will appeal to the entire family. (In case you're curious, the Altrurians are a club group at whose meeting I first "tasted" a soup like this with my eyes!)   ☻   Serves 4 (1½ cups)

> 2¾ cups water
> 1½ cups (8 ounces) diced cooked lean roast beef
> 3 cups sliced carrots
> 1 cup chopped celery
> ½ cup chopped onion
> ¼ teaspoon black pepper
> 1 teaspoon dried parsley flakes
> 1¾ cups (3 ounces) uncooked wide noodles
> 1 (12-ounce) jar Heinz Fat Free Beef Gravy

In a large saucepan, combine water, roast beef, carrots, celery, onion, black pepper, and parsley flakes. Bring mixture to a boil. Lower heat, cover, and simmer for 20 minutes. Stir in uncooked noodles and gravy. Continue simmering for 10 minutes or until vegetables and noodles are tender, stirring occasionally.

HINTS: 1. Even better reheated the next day.
2. If you don't have leftovers, purchase a chunk of cooked lean roast beef from your local deli.

Each serving equals:

HE: 2¼ Vegetable • 2 Protein • 1 Bread • ¼ Slider • 18 Optional Calories

---

273 Calories • 5 gm Fat • 22 gm Protein • 35 gm Carbohydrate • 595 mg Sodium • 53 mg Calcium • 4 gm Fiber

---

DIABETIC: 2 Vegetable • 2 Meat • 1 Starch

Rotini Ham Soup

My husband, Cliff, inspires many of my recipes, including this one that invites some of his favorite foods to shake hands and say "howdy!" Preparing the tomato soup with milk lets me sneak in a little healthy calcium, and stirring in all those tasty bits of ham gives this some real man-pleasing flavor!

● Serves 4 (full 1¼ cups)

1 (10¾-ounce) can Healthy Request Tomato Soup
1⅓ cups skim milk
1 teaspoon dried onion flakes
1 teaspoon dried parsley flakes
1 teaspoon Italian seasoning
2 cups (one 16-ounce can) cut green beans, rinsed and drained
1 full cup (6 ounces) diced Dubuque 97% fat-free ham or any
    extra-lean ham
2 cups hot cooked rotini pasta, rinsed and drained
¼ cup (¾ ounce) grated Kraft fat-free Parmesan cheese

In a large saucepan, combine tomato soup, skim milk, onion flakes, parsley flakes, and Italian seasoning. Stir in green beans, ham, and rotini pasta. Bring mixture to a boil. Lower heat, cover, and simmer for 10 minutes, stirring occasionally. When serving, top each bowl with 1 tablespoon Parmesan cheese.

HINT: 1½ cups uncooked rotini pasta usually cooks to about 2 cups.

Each serving equals:

HE: 1¼ Protein • 1 Bread • ½ Vegetable •
⅓ Skim Milk • ½ Slider • 5 Optional Calories

251 Calories • 3 gm Fat • 15 gm Protein •
41 gm Carbohydrate • 747 mg Sodium •
133 mg Calcium • 3 gm Fiber

DIABETIC: 2 Starch • 1½ Meat • 1 Vegetable

Hamburger Tomato Rice Soup

I like to layer flavors sometimes, as I have in this recipe, blending tomato soup and sauce for a delicious intensity. Anyone sipping this soup might wonder if you've simply harvested your tomato patch right into the pot! ☻ Serves 4 (1½ cups)

> 8 ounces ground 90% lean turkey or beef
> ½ cup chopped onion
> 1 (10¾-ounce) can Healthy Request Tomato Soup
> 1¾ cups (one 15-ounce can) Hunt's Tomato Sauce
> 2 cups water
> ⅔ cup (1½ ounces) uncooked Minute Rice
> 1 teaspoon dried parsley flakes
> ⅛ teaspoon black pepper

In a large saucepan sprayed with butter-flavored cooking spray, brown meat and onion. Stir in tomato soup, tomato sauce, and water. Bring mixture to a boil. Add rice, parsley flakes, and black pepper. Mix well to combine. Lower heat, cover, and simmer for 10 minutes, stirring occasionally.

Each serving equals:

HE: 2 Vegetable • 1½ Protein • ½ Bread • ½ Slider • 5 Optional Calories

190 Calories • 6 gm Fat • 12 gm Protein • 22 gm Carbohydrate • 985 mg Sodium • 16 mg Calcium • 3 gm Fiber

DIABETIC: 1½ Vegetable • 1½ Meat • 1 Starch

Vegetables

Vegetable Platter

Some "diet" cookbooks might suggest cutting up lots of fresh veggies to snack on, but all that raw crunch may not set everyone's taste buds to humming. Here's a flavorful trick to make that veggie "buffet" outrageously delicious and tangy with hardly any effort.

◐ Serves 4

> *2 cups fresh broccoli pieces*
> *2 cups fresh cauliflower pieces*
> *2 cups sliced unpeeled zucchini*
> *2 cups peeled and chopped fresh tomatoes*
> *¼ cup Kraft Fat Free Italian Dressing*
> *¼ cup (¾ ounce) grated Kraft fat-free Parmesan cheese*

Place broccoli, cauliflower, and zucchini in an 8-by-8-inch glass baking dish. Cover and microwave on HIGH (100% power) for 9 to 10 minutes. Drain off moisture, if necessary. Add tomatoes. Mix gently to combine. Drizzle Italian dressing over vegetables. Sprinkle Parmesan cheese evenly over top. Re-cover and microwave on HIGH for 3 minutes. Let set for 1 to 2 minutes. Divide into 4 servings.

Each serving equals:

HE: 4 Vegetable • ¼ Protein • 4 Optional Calories

---

80 Calories • 0 gm Fat • 4 gm Protein •
16 gm Carbohydrate • 272 mg Sodium •
46 mg Calcium • 5 gm Fiber

DIABETIC: 3 Vegetable

Creamy Vegetable Medley

Isn't there something extra-cozy about serving vegetables in a rich cream sauce? It's the kind of dish you'd serve to company on a festive occasion, but why save it just for that? Here's an utterly quick and easy "party" dish that makes any meal a celebration.

● Serves 4 (1 cup)

> 1 (10¾-ounce) can Healthy Request Cream of Celery Soup
> ⅓ cup skim milk
> ½ teaspoon lemon pepper
> 4 cups frozen cauliflower, broccoli, and carrot blend, thawed

In a large skillet sprayed with butter-flavored cooking spray, combine celery soup, skim milk, and lemon pepper. Add vegetables. Mix well to combine. Cook over medium heat for 10 minutes, or until mixture is heated through, stirring occasionally.

HINT: Thaw vegetables by placing in a colander and rinsing under hot water for one minute.

Each serving equals:

> HE: 2 Vegetable • ½ Slider • 9 Optional Calories
>
> ---
> 89 Calories • 1 gm Fat • 4 gm Protein •
> 16 gm Carbohydrate • 356 mg Sodium •
> 123 mg Calcium • 3 gm Fiber
>
> ---
> DIABETIC: 2 Vegetable • ½ Starch

Scalloped Cabbage and Mushrooms

This dish may sound a bit unusual, but I think you'll be pleasantly surprised by this captivating combo of textures and tastes! It's healthy (lots of fiber and calcium), and simple to stir up. Best of all, it fills your tummy and satisfies your soul!　●　Serves 4

> 1 (10¾-ounce) can Healthy Request Cream of Mushroom Soup
> ½ cup skim milk
> ¾ cup (3 ounces) shredded Kraft reduced-fat Cheddar cheese
> 2 teaspoons dried onion flakes
> ½ cup (one 2.5-ounce jar) sliced mushrooms, undrained
> 4 cups shredded cabbage

Preheat oven to 350 degrees. Spray an 8-by-8-inch baking dish with butter-flavored cooking spray. In a large skillet sprayed with butter-flavored cooking spray, combine mushroom soup, skim milk, Cheddar cheese, onion flakes, and undrained mushrooms. Cook over medium heat until sauce thickens and cheese melts, stirring often. Add cabbage. Mix well to combine. Lower heat and simmer for 5 minutes, stirring occasionally. Spread cabbage mixture into prepared baking dish. Cover and bake for 1 hour. Uncover and continue baking for 15 minutes. Divide into 4 servings.

Each serving equals:

> HE: 2¼ Vegetable • 1 Protein • ½ Slider •
> 12 Optional Calories
>
> ---
>
> 133 Calories • 5 gm Fat • 8 gm Protein •
> 14 gm Carbohydrate • 590 mg Sodium •
> 264 mg Calcium • 2 gm Fiber
>
> ---
>
> DIABETIC: 1 Vegetable • 1 Meat • ½ Starch

Quick Creole Green Beans

I can save you a flight to New Orleans with this tangy veggie sauté! This sweet-and-tangy blend of green beans and tomatoes offers a culinary side trip to Louisiana for lunch.

Serves 6 (1 cup)

¼ cup chopped onion

2 tablespoons Hormel Bacon Bits

1¾ cups (one 14½-ounce can) stewed tomatoes, undrained

1 tablespoon Sugar Twin or Sprinkle Sweet

4 cups (two 16-ounce cans) cut green beans, rinsed and drained

In a large skillet sprayed with butter-flavored cooking spray, sauté onion for 5 minutes or until tender. Stir in bacon bits, undrained stewed tomatoes, and Sugar Twin. Add green beans. Mix well to combine. Lower heat, cover, and simmer for 5 minutes, or until mixture is heated through, stirring occasionally.

Each serving equals:

HE: 2 Vegetable • 9 Optional Calories

48 Calories • 0 gm Fat • 3 gm Protein • 9 gm Carbohydrate • 295 mg Sodium • 62 mg Calcium • 2 gm Fiber

DIABETIC: 2 Vegetable

Green Beans and Mushroom Medley

They say it takes two to tango, and it's also true that two can be lots better than one when it comes to lip-smacking flavor! This is a great side dish to stir up fast when unexpected company comes for dinner. It's colorful, it tastes great, and is completely fat-free!

◐ Serves 6 (¾ cup)

½ cup chopped onion

½ cup Kraft Fat Free Italian Dressing

4 cups (two 16-ounce cans) cut green beans, rinsed and drained

½ cup (one 2.5-ounce jar) sliced mushrooms, drained

¼ cup (one 2-ounce jar) chopped pimiento, drained

1 tablespoon Sugar Twin or Sprinkle Sweet

In a large skillet sprayed with olive oil–flavored cooking spray, sauté onion for 5 minutes or until tender. Stir in Italian dressing. Add green beans, mushrooms, pimiento, and Sugar Twin. Mix well to combine. Lower heat and simmer for 5 minutes, stirring occasionally.

Each serving equals:

HE: 1⅔ Vegetable • 6 Optional Calories

36 Calories • 0 gm Fat • 1 gm Protein •
8 gm Carbohydrate • 265 mg Sodium •
28 mg Calcium • 2 gm Fiber

DIABETIC: 1½ Vegetable

Skillet Green Beans

Here's another "Cliff-pleaser"—it's true, the man just can't get enough green beans! He also loves finding those bits of bacon and onion as he gobbles down every last one.

● Serves 4 (¾ cup)

> 1 (10¾-ounce) can Healthy Request Tomato Soup
> ¼ cup water
> 2 tablespoons Hormel Bacon Bits
> 1 teaspoon dried onion flakes
> 4 cups (two 16-ounce cans) cut green beans, rinsed and drained

In a large skillet, combine tomato soup, water, bacon bits, and onion flakes. Bring mixture to a boil. Stir in green beans. Lower heat and simmer for 5 minutes, or until mixture is heated through, stirring occasionally.

Each serving equals:

HE: 2 Vegetable • ¾ Slider • 3 Optional Calories

89 Calories • 1 gm Fat • 4 gm Protein •
16 gm Carbohydrate • 358 mg Sodium •
44 mg Calcium • 2 gm Fiber

DIABETIC: 2 Vegetable • ½ Starch

Home on the Range Beans

This side dish is so filling and high in protein, it may give you a whole new appreciation of eating vegetarian! On cattle drives, nothing could be tastier than the pot of beans that simmered for hours over a campfire. This dish takes a fraction of the time, but it'll still inspire the cowboys in your house to smack their lips.

☻ Serves 6 (scant 1 cup)

> ½ cup chopped onion
> ½ cup chopped green bell pepper
> 1 cup (one 8-ounce can) Hunt's Tomato Sauce
> 2 tablespoons Brown Sugar Twin
> 2 tablespoons Sugar Twin or Sprinkle Sweet
> 1 teaspoon prepared mustard
> 1 tablespoon white vinegar
> 2 teaspoons chili seasoning
> 10 ounces (one 16-ounce can) pinto beans, rinsed and drained
> 10 ounces (one 16-ounce can) red kidney beans, rinsed and drained
> 10 ounces (one 16-ounce can) butter or lima beans, rinsed and
>   drained

In a large skillet sprayed with butter-flavored cooking spray, sauté onion and green pepper for 5 minutes or until tender. Stir in tomato sauce, Brown Sugar Twin, Sugar Twin, mustard, vinegar, and chili seasoning. Add pinto beans, kidney beans, and butter beans. Mix well to combine. Lower heat, cover, and simmer for 10 minutes, stirring occasionally.

Each serving equals:

HE: 2½ Protein • 1 Vegetable • 4 Optional Calories

153 Calories • 1 gm Fat • 8 gm Protein •
28 gm Carbohydrate • 476 mg Sodium •
62 mg Calcium • 8 gm Fiber

DIABETIC: 1½ Starch • 1 Meat • 1 Vegetable

Grandma's Carrots

When I first tasted this dish, it brought me back to my childhood and recalled the rich, old-fashioned flavor of vegetables served at my grandmother's boardinghouse table. This is a wonderful way to serve up your garden's healthy harvest and savor the sweet abundance along with the memories. ☻ Serves 6 (¾ cup)

1 cup chopped onion

5 cups fresh or frozen cut carrots

*2 tablespoons chopped fresh parsley or 2 teaspoons dried parsley
    flakes*

1¾ cups (one 15-ounce can) Swanson Beef Broth

1 (10¾-ounce) can Healthy Request Cream of Mushroom Soup

In a large skillet sprayed with butter-flavored cooking spray, sauté onion for 5 minutes or until tender. Add carrots, parsley, and beef broth. Mix well to combine. Cover and cook over medium heat for 20 minutes. Uncover, and stir in mushroom soup. Continue cooking for 10 to 12 minutes or until carrots are tender. Serve at once.

Each serving equals:

HE: 2 Vegetable • ¼ Slider • 13 Optional Calories

81 Calories • 1 gm Fat • 2 gm Protein •
16 gm Carbohydrate • 473 mg Sodium •
66 mg Calcium • 3 gm Fiber

DIABETIC: 2 Vegetable • ½ Starch

Braised Celery and Carrots

This oven-baked combination produces an astonishingly succulent side dish so full of fiber you'll feel healthier just munching away! If you're stuck in the rut of eating raw carrots and celery all the time, why not try something new with these classic veggies? I bet you'll make this recipe one of your newest favorites!

♥ Serves 6

> 3 cups coarsely chopped celery
> 3 cups coarsely chopped carrots
> 2 cups water
> 1 cup sliced onion
> 1¾ cups (one 15-ounce can) Swanson Beef Broth
> 3 tablespoons all-purpose flour
> 1 teaspoon dried parsley flakes

Preheat oven to 350 degrees. Spray an 8-by-8-inch baking dish with butter-flavored cooking spray. In a medium saucepan, cook celery and carrots in water for 10 minutes. Add onion. Mix well to combine. Continue cooking vegetables for 5 minutes. Drain and place partially cooked hot vegetables in prepared baking dish. In a covered jar, combine beef broth, flour, and parsley flakes. Shake well to blend. Pour broth mixture into a medium saucepan sprayed with butter-flavored cooking spray. Cook over medium heat until mixture thickens, stirring often. Pour hot broth mixture over vegetables. Cover and bake for 45 minutes. Uncover and continue baking for 15 minutes. Divide into 6 servings. Serve at once.

Each serving equals:

HE: 3½ Vegetable • ¼ Slider • 1 Optional Calorie

---

60 Calories • 0 gm Fat • 2 gm Protein •
13 gm Carbohydrate • 312 mg Sodium •
46 mg Calcium • 3 gm Fiber

DIABETIC: 3 Vegetable

BBQ Corn and Tomato Sauté

Here's an amazing example of how one ingredient can transform a dish into party food! Just tumble all these veggies into a skillet, then add the Brown Sugar Twin, and *voilà!* Your mouth will be convinced you fired up the grill! ● Serves 4 (¾ cup)

> ¼ cup chopped onion
> ¼ cup chopped green bell pepper
> 1 cup peeled and chopped fresh tomatoes
> 2 tablespoons Brown Sugar Twin
> 2 cups (one 16-ounce can) whole-kernel corn, rinsed and drained

In a large skillet sprayed with butter-flavored cooking spray, sauté onion, green pepper, and tomatoes for 5 minutes. Stir in Brown Sugar Twin and corn. Lower heat and simmer for 5 minutes, stirring occasionally.

Each serving equals:

HE: 1 Bread • ¾ Vegetable • 2 Optional Calories

92 Calories • 0 gm Fat • 3 gm Protein •
20 gm Carbohydrate • 9 mg Sodium • 6 mg Calcium •
3 gm Fiber

DIABETIC: 1 Starch • 1 Vegetable

Boston Baked Corn

Sometimes your mind plays culinary tricks, as it did on me with this dish. I was thinking of that old-fashioned American classic, Boston baked beans . . . and then I wondered, *mmm,* what about cooking up a pot of corn flavored in just that way? This is the finger-lickin'-good result, and it's a wow!

○ Serves 6 (½ cup)

> 1 cup (one 8-ounce can) Hunt's Tomato Sauce
>
> 1 tablespoon Brown Sugar Twin
>
> 1 teaspoon prepared mustard
>
> 1 teaspoon dried parsley flakes
>
> ½ cup chopped onion
>
> ½ cup chopped green bell pepper
>
> 3 cups frozen whole-kernel corn, thawed
>
> 2 tablespoons Hormel Bacon Bits

In a slow cooker container, combine tomato sauce, Brown Sugar Twin, mustard, and parsley flakes. Add onion, green pepper, and corn. Mix well to combine. Stir in bacon bits. Cover and cook on LOW for 6 to 8 hours. Mix well before serving.

HINT: Thaw corn by placing in a colander and rinsing under hot water for one minute.

Each serving equals:

HE: 1 Vegetable • 1 Bread • 10 Optional Calories

100 Calories • 0 gm Fat • 4 gm Protein •
21 gm Carbohydrate • 366 mg Sodium •
7 mg Calcium • 3 gm Fiber

DIABETIC: 1 Vegetable • 1 Starch

Peas with Dill

If you're not in the habit of cooking with dill, I hope you'll take my hand and "jump in" with this recipe! Just a tiny amount of this savory herb takes a bowl of everyday peas into a new dimension. You may decide someday to grow a little dill in your window box garden, but in the meantime, the dried version tastes just fine.

○ Serves 4 (½ cup)

¼ cup chopped onion

2 cups frozen peas, thawed

¼ cup (one 2-ounce jar) chopped pimiento, drained

½ teaspoon dried dill weed

2 teaspoons reduced-calorie margarine

In a large skillet sprayed with butter-flavored cooking spray, sauté onion for 5 minutes or until tender. Add peas, pimiento, dill weed, and margarine. Mix well to combine. Lower heat, cover, and simmer for 2 to 3 minutes, or until mixture is heated through. Serve at once.

HINT: Thaw peas by placing in a colander and rinsing under hot water for one minute.

Each serving equals:

HE: 1 Bread • ¼ Vegetable • ¼ Fat

73 Calories • 1 gm Fat • 4 gm Protein •
12 gm Carbohydrate • 15 mg Sodium •
23 mg Calcium • 4 gm Fiber

DIABETIC: 1 Starch

Barbecued Kraut

Cliff and I enjoy sauerkraut so much, I'm always on the lookout for fun new ways to serve this favorite. We both voted "Aye" on this tangy, slow-cooked version that's smoky and sweet!

❂ Serves 6 (¾ cup)

> 1 cup (one 8-ounce can) Hunt's Tomato Sauce
> 2 tablespoons Brown Sugar Twin
> 2 tablespoons Sugar Twin or Sprinkle Sweet
> 1 teaspoon Worcestershire sauce
> ¼ cup Hormel Bacon Bits
> ½ cup finely chopped onion
> 3½ cups (two 14½-ounce cans) Frank's Bavarian-style sauer-
>   kraut, drained

In a slow cooker container, combine tomato sauce, Brown Sugar Twin, Sugar Twin, and Worcestershire sauce. Stir in bacon bits and onion. Add sauerkraut. Mix well to combine. Cover and cook on LOW for 6 to 8 hours. Mix well before serving.

HINT: If you can't find Bavarian sauerkraut, use regular sauerkraut, ½ teaspoon caraway seeds, and 1 teaspoon Brown
Sugar Twin.

Each serving equals:

HE: 2 Vegetable • ¼ Slider • 1 Optional Calorie

---

65 Calories • 1 gm Fat • 4 gm Protein •
10 gm Carbohydrate • 1,352 mg Sodium •
45 mg Calcium • 4 gm Fiber

DIABETIC: 2 Vegetable

Stuffed Harvest Squash

This looks pretty enough to grace your Thanksgiving table, and it smells so utterly delicious you'll be seeing hungry faces at your kitchen door long before dinner is ready! Most of my recipes can be served all year round, but this one just seems to cry out for a crisp fall evening when the leaves are every shade of gold and red!

○ Serves 4

1 cup (2 small) cored, unpeeled, and chopped cooking apples

¼ cup raisins

2 tablespoons Brown Sugar Twin

¼ teaspoon apple pie spice

2 small (about 16 ounces each) acorn squash

In a small bowl, combine apples, raisins, Brown Sugar Twin, and apple pie spice. Cut each squash in half. Scoop out and discard seeds and membrane. Evenly stuff each half with about ⅓ cup apple mixture. Place squash in a 9-by-13-inch glass baking dish. Cover and microwave on HIGH (100% power) for 12 minutes, turning dish after 6 minutes. Uncover and lightly spray tops with butter-flavored cooking spray. Continue to microwave on HIGH for 2 minutes. Let set for 2 to 3 minutes before serving.

Each serving equals:

HE: 1½ Starch • 1 Fruit • 2 Optional Calories

168 Calories • 0 gm Fat • 0 gm Protein •
42 gm Carbohydrate • 5 mg Sodium •
56 mg Calcium • 6 gm Fiber

DIABETIC: 1½ Starch • 1 Fruit

Zucchini Patties

Everyone loves to joke about the overabundance of end-of-season zucchini, but if this tasty green squash is piling up in your pantry and you can't make room for another loaf of zucchini bread, here's a new way to relish this veggie! I've suggested this as a side dish, but if your family likes it as much as mine did, it's a good choice for a meatless main dish too. ◐   Serves 6

> 2 cups shredded unpeeled zucchini
> 6 tablespoons Bisquick Reduced Fat Baking Mix
> ¼ cup (¾ ounce) grated Kraft fat-free Parmesan cheese
> ⅓ cup (1½ ounces) shredded Kraft reduced-fat Cheddar cheese
> 2 teaspoons dried onion flakes
> ½ teaspoon lemon pepper
> 1 egg, slightly beaten, or equivalent in egg substitute
> 3 tablespoons Kraft Fat Free Italian Dressing

In a large bowl, combine zucchini, baking mix, Parmesan cheese, Cheddar cheese, onion flakes, and lemon pepper. Add egg. Mix well to combine. Pour Italian dressing into a large skillet and heat until dressing is warm. Using a ¼-cup measuring cup as a guide, form zucchini mix into 6 patties and evenly arrange patties in skillet. Cook over medium low heat for 4 to 5 minutes on each side or until lightly browned. Serve warm.

Each serving equals:

HE: ⅔ Vegetable • ⅔ Protein • ⅓ Bread • 2 Optional Calories

74 Calories • 2 gm Fat • 4 gm Protein • 10 gm Carbohydrate • 289 mg Sodium • 64 mg Calcium • 1 gm Fiber

DIABETIC: 1 Meat • ½ Starch/Carbohydrate

Zucchini-Stuffed Potatoes

This high-fiber filling for baked potatoes abounds with creamy, cheesy goodness and provides lots of good nutrition too! Once you taste it, you'll find it hard to believe that this scrumptious dish has *zero* fat grams—it tastes absolutely decadent!   ☻   Serves 4

> *4 medium (5 ounces each) baking potatoes*
> *⅔ cup Carnation Nonfat Dry Milk Powder*
> *½ cup water*
> *¼ cup Kraft Fat Free Italian Dressing*
> *1 cup grated unpeeled zucchini*
> *¼ cup (¾ ounce) grated Kraft fat-free Parmesan cheese*
> *Dash paprika*

Bake potatoes until tender. Cut each potato in half lengthwise. Scoop potato pulp into a large bowl, reserving shells. Mash potato pulp with potato masher or fork. Add dry milk powder and water. Mix well to combine. Set aside. In a large skillet, combine Italian dressing and zucchini. Cook over medium heat for about 5 minutes, or until zucchini is tender, stirring often. Add hot zucchini mixture and Parmesan cheese to potato mixture. Mix well to combine. Evenly spoon mixture into reserved potato shells. Place stuffed potatoes in a 9-by-13-inch baking dish. Lightly sprinkle paprika over top. Bake at 350 degrees for 10 minutes. Lightly spray tops with butter-flavored cooking spray. Serve at once.

Each serving equals:

HE: 1 Bread • ½ Skim Milk • ½ Vegetable • ¼ Protein • 4 Optional Calories

---

188 Calories • 0 gm Fat • 7 gm Protein • 40 gm Carbohydrate • 303 mg Sodium • 150 mg Calcium • 3 gm Fiber

---

DIABETIC: 2 Starch • ½ Skim Milk

Farmhouse Skillet Potatoes

Sometimes you just want a quick and tasty stovetop potato dish, and this one truly fits the bill! Cliff loved the combo of green beans with potatoes, and he commented that the blend of two peppers gave it lots of extra flavor. ☻ Serves 4 (1 full cup)

4 cups (20 ounces) thinly sliced unpeeled raw potatoes
1 cup diced onion
2 cups (one 16-ounce can) cut green beans, drained, and ½ cup
    liquid reserved
½ teaspoon lemon pepper
¼ teaspoon black pepper

In a large skillet sprayed with butter-flavored cooking spray, combine potatoes and onion. Cover and cook over medium-low heat for 5 minutes, stirring occasionally. Add green beans, reserved liquid, lemon pepper, and black pepper. Mix well to combine. Re-cover and continue simmering for 10 minutes, stirring occasionally. Serve at once.

HINT: Good topped with 1 tablespoon fat-free sour cream.

Each serving equals:

HE: 1½ Vegetable • 1 Bread

116 Calories • 0 gm Fat • 3 gm Protein •
26 gm Carbohydrate • 79 mg Sodium •
36 mg Calcium • 3 gm Fiber

DIABETIC: 1 Starch • 1 Vegetable

New Age Scalloped Potatoes

If the microwave did nothing else but cook potatoes fast and fla-
vorfully, I'd make room for it in my tiny home kitchen! (And of
course, it does much more. . . .) This recipe delivers wonderfully
tender potatoes in a creamy mushroom-cheese sauce that is simply
irresistible!   ☻   Serves 4

> ¾ cup water
> ⅓ cup Carnation Nonfat Dry Milk Powder
> 1 (10¾-ounce) can Healthy Request Cream of Mushroom Soup
> 4 cups (20 ounces) sliced raw potatoes
> ¾ cup (3 ounces) shredded Kraft reduced-fat Cheddar cheese
> ½ cup finely chopped onion
> 1 teaspoon dried parsley flakes

In an 8-by-8-inch glass baking dish, combine water, dry milk
powder, and mushroom soup. Stir in potatoes, Cheddar cheese,
onion, and parsley flakes. Cover and microwave on HIGH (100%
power) for 10 minutes. Uncover and stir. Re-cover and continue to
microwave on HIGH for 10 to 12 minutes or until potatoes are tender. Place baking dish on a wire rack and let set 5 minutes. Divide
into 4 servings.

Each serving equals:

HE: 1 Bread • 1 Protein • ¼ Skim Milk •
¼ Vegetable • ½ Slider • 1 Optional Calorie

209 Calories • 5 gm Fat • 10 gm Protein •
31 gm Carbohydrate • 517 mg Sodium •
274 mg Calcium • 2 gm Fiber

DIABETIC: 2 Starch • 1 Protein

Savory Salads

Wilted Greens Salad

It sounds a little odd, doesn't it, to prepare a salad where the greens are wilted. But trust me, when you wilt the greens deliberately by tossing them with a hot and tangy dressing, you'll be surprised just how delectable a funny-sounding dish can taste!

☻ Serves 4 (1¼ cups)

> 4 cups torn leaf lettuce or spinach, stems discarded
> ¾ cup sliced fresh mushrooms
> ¼ cup sliced green onion
> ¼ cup white vinegar
> 1 tablespoon Sugar Twin or Sprinkle Sweet
> ½ teaspoon prepared mustard
> 2 tablespoons Hormel Bacon Bits

In a large bowl, combine lettuce, mushrooms, and onion. In a large skillet sprayed with butter-flavored cooking spray, combine vinegar, Sugar Twin, and mustard. Add bacon bits. Mix well to combine. Bring mixture to a boil. Pour hot mixture over lettuce mixture. Toss lightly to coat. Serve at once.

Each serving equals:

HE: 2½ Vegetable • 14 Optional Calories

---

33 Calories • 1 gm Fat • 2 gm Protein •
4 gm Carbohydrate • 139 mg Sodium •
15 mg Calcium • 1 gm Fiber

DIABETIC: 1 Vegetable

Thousand Island Garden Salad

Of course, you could serve plain old Thousand Island dressing straight from the bottle over hearts of lettuce, but it takes so little extra effort to make what's ordinary—extraordinary! This creamy concoction is wonderfully crunchy and creamy all at once.

◗ Serves 4 (⅔ cup)

1 cup sliced unpeeled cucumbers
1 cup chopped fresh tomatoes
¼ cup sliced radishes
½ cup chopped celery
¼ cup chopped green bell pepper
¼ cup Kraft fat-free mayonnaise
¼ cup Kraft Fat Free Thousand Island Dressing
2 tablespoons Hormel Bacon Bits
1 teaspoon dried parsley flakes

In a medium bowl, combine cucumbers, tomatoes, radishes, celery, and green pepper. In a small bowl, combine mayonnaise, Thousand Island dressing, bacon bits, and parsley flakes. Add mayonnaise mixture to vegetable mixture. Mix gently to combine. Cover and refrigerate for at least 15 minutes. Gently stir again just before serving.

Each serving equals:

HE: 1½ Vegetable • ½ Slider • 8 Optional Calories

65 Calories • 1 gm Fat • 2 gm Protein •
12 gm Carbohydrate • 415 mg Sodium •
16 mg Calcium • 2 gm Fiber

DIABETIC: 2 Vegetable *or*
1½ Vegetable • ½ Starch/Carbohydrate

Continental Cucumber Garden Salad

When a country shares a border with another country, the two may not always get along. But here's one way Italy and France make beautiful music together—in this flavorful chopped salad dressed with the best of both! ☻ Serves 6 (⅔ cup)

> *2 cups sliced unpeeled cucumbers*
> *¼ cup chopped onion*
> *¼ cup chopped green bell pepper*
> *1½ cups chopped fresh tomatoes*
> *2 tablespoons Hormel Bacon Bits*
> *¼ cup Kraft Fat Free Italian Dressing*
> *¼ cup Kraft Fat Free French Dressing*

In a large bowl, combine cucumbers, onion, green pepper, tomatoes, and bacon bits. Add Italian dressing and French dressing. Mix gently to combine. Cover and refrigerate for at least 30 minutes. Gently stir again just before serving.

Each serving equals:

HE: 1⅓ Vegetable • 14 Optional Calories

44 Calories • 0 gm Fat • 2 gm Protein •
9 gm Carbohydrate • 292 mg Sodium •
9 mg Calcium • 1 gm Fiber

DIABETIC: 1½ Vegetable

Carrot-Peanut-Apple Salad

Sweet and salty, crunchy and creamy—and all at the same time! That's the scrumptious secret of this salad that just overflows with goodness. It's also attractively colorful and makes a lovely dish for a harvest-time buffet.   ☻   Serves 6 (⅔ cup)

> 2 cups shredded carrots
> 1½ cups (3 small) cored, unpeeled, and chopped Red Delicious
>   apples
> 6 tablespoons raisins
> ¼ cup (1 ounce) chopped dry-roasted peanuts
> ⅓ cup Kraft fat-free mayonnaise
> 2 tablespoons skim milk
> 2 tablespoons Peter Pan reduced-fat peanut butter

In a large bowl, combine carrots, apples, raisins, and peanuts. In a small bowl, combine mayonnaise, skim milk, and peanut butter. Mix well until smooth. Add mayonnaise mixture to carrot mixture. Mix well to combine. Cover and refrigerate for at least 15 minutes. Gently stir again just before serving.

HINT: To plump up raisins without "cooking," place in a glass
    measuring cup and microwave on HIGH for 15 to 20 seconds.

Each serving equals:

HE: 1 Fruit • ⅔ Vegetable • ⅔ Fat • ½ Protein •
11 Optional Calories

128 Calories • 4 gm Fat • 3 gm Protein •
20 gm Carbohydrate • 133 mg Sodium •
26 mg Calcium • 2 gm Fiber

DIABETIC: 1 Fruit • ½ Starch • ½ Fat

Nadine's Creamy Orange Vegetable Salad

This pretty blend tastes as good as it looks—and it looks like a perfect sunset after a sunny summer day! I always think a dish should feed the eye as well as the tummy, and this one does both with pizazz. ☻ Serves 8

> 2 (4-serving) packages JELL-O sugar-free orange gelatin
> 1 cup boiling water
> ¾ cup cold water
> 1 cup Kraft fat-free mayonnaise
> 2 cups fat-free cottage cheese
> 1½ cups shredded carrots
> 1 cup finely chopped celery
> ¼ cup finely chopped onion
> ¼ cup finely chopped green bell pepper

In a large bowl, combine dry gelatin and boiling water. Mix well to dissolve gelatin. Stir in cold water and mayonnaise. Fold in cottage cheese. Add carrots, celery, onion, and green pepper. Mix gently to combine. Pour mixture into a 9-by-13-inch cake pan. Refrigerate until firm, about 3 hours. Cut into 8 servings.

Each serving equals:

HE: ¾ Vegetable • ½ Protein • ¼ Slider •
10 Optional Calories

---

80 Calories • 0 gm Fat • 9 gm Protein •
11 gm Carbohydrate • 546 mg Sodium •
37 mg Calcium • 1 gm Fiber

DIABETIC: 1 Vegetable • ½ Meat • ½ Starch

Holiday Slaw

Fruity and nutty, this luscious side dish is wonderful for so many special occasions. It's such an inventive blend of tastes and textures, your guests will be intrigued by every single bite!

○ Serves 6 (⅔ cup)

> 2 cups shredded cabbage
> 2 cups (2 medium) diced bananas
> 1 cup (one 8-ounce can) crushed pineapple, packed in fruit juice,
>   drained
> 4 maraschino cherries, diced
> ¼ cup (1 ounce) chopped pecans
> ½ cup (1 ounce) miniature marshmallows
> ¼ cup Kraft fat-free mayonnaise
> ½ cup Cool Whip Free

In a medium bowl, combine cabbage, bananas, pineapple, maraschino cherries, pecans, and marshmallows. In a small bowl, combine mayonnaise and Cool Whip Free. Add mayonnaise mixture to cabbage mixture. Mix gently to combine. Cover and refrigerate for at least 1 hour. Gently stir again just before serving.

HINT: To prevent bananas from turning brown, mix with 1 teaspoon lemon juice or sprinkle with Fruit Fresh.

Each serving equals:

HE: 1 Fruit • ⅔ Vegetable • ⅔ Fat • ¼ Slider •
15 Optional Calories

---

139 Calories • 3 gm Fat • 1 gm Protein •
27 gm Carbohydrate • 97 mg Sodium •
22 mg Calcium • 2 gm Fiber

DIABETIC: 1 Fruit • 1 Fat • ½ Carbohydrate/Starch

Honey Slaw Salad

I'm such a big fan of coleslaw, I've probably created dozens of coleslaw recipes over the years. Now, by stirring a couple of tablespoons of my absolutely favorite nuts into the mix, along with a sweet and tangy dressing, I've found my new number 1!

☻ Serves 4 (full ¾ cup)

> 2½ cups purchased coleslaw mix
> 2 tablespoons (½ ounce) chopped pecans
> ⅓ cup Land O Lakes no-fat sour cream
> ¼ cup Kraft Fat Free Honey Dijon Dressing

In a large bowl, combine coleslaw mix and pecans. In a small bowl, combine sour cream and Honey Dijon dressing. Add sour cream mixture to coleslaw mixture. Mix well to combine. Cover and refrigerate for at least 30 minutes. Gently stir again just before serving.

HINT: 2 cups shredded cabbage and ½ cup shredded carrots may be used in place of purchased coleslaw mix.

Each serving equals:

HE: 1¼ Vegetable • ½ Fat • ¼ Slider •
12 Optional Calories

82 Calories • 2 gm Fat • 2 gm Protein •
14 gm Carbohydrate • 206 mg Sodium •
42 mg Calcium • 2 gm Fiber

DIABETIC: 1 Vegetable • ½ Starch • ½ Fat

Grandpa's Creamy Coleslaw

When I watch Cliff with our grandbabies, I sometimes marvel that a man so young in spirit can actually be a grandpa! I surely had him in mind when I mixed up this coleslaw just brimming with old-timey taste—the kind that memories are made of. (If you're ever passing through DeWitt, Iowa, stop by my cafe for a taste of this—it's always on the menu!) ☻ Serves 4 (¾ cup)

3½ cups purchased coleslaw mix
¾ cup diced celery
¼ cup chopped onion
⅔ cup Kraft fat-free mayonnaise
Sugar substitute to equal 1 tablespoon sugar
1 tablespoon white vinegar
1 tablespoon Dijon Country Style mustard
1 tablespoon dried parsley flakes
⅛ teaspoon black pepper

In a large bowl, combine coleslaw mix, celery, and onion. In a small bowl, combine mayonnaise, sugar substitute, vinegar, mustard, parsley flakes, and black pepper. Add mayonnaise mixture to cabbage mixture. Mix well to combine. Cover and refrigerate for at least 30 minutes. Gently stir again just before serving.

HINT: 2¾ cups shredded cabbage and ¾ cup shredded carrots may be used in place of purchased coleslaw mix.

Each serving equals:

HE: 2¼ Vegetable • ¼ Slider • 8 Optional Calories

64 Calories • 0 gm Fat • 2 gm Protein •
14 gm Carbohydrate • 472 mg Sodium •
44 mg Calcium • 2 gm Fiber

DIABETIC: 2 Vegetable

Grandma's Potato Salad

Everyone's grandma used to have her own secret recipe for potato salad, and I'm sure no family's summer potluck was complete without a couple of these beloved dishes. This classic blend couldn't be easier to fix, but I bet your own grandma would be proud to taste it. It's a mainstay at JO's Kitchen Cafe every single day!

◑ Serves 4 (full ¾ cup)

> 2½ cups (12 ounces) diced cooked potatoes
> ¾ cup diced celery
> ¼ cup chopped onion
> ⅔ cup Kraft fat-free mayonnaise
> Sugar substitute to equal 1 tablespoon sugar
> 1 tablespoon white vinegar
> 1 tablespoon Dijon Country Style mustard
> 1 tablespoon dried parsley flakes
> ⅛ teaspoon black pepper
> 1 hard-boiled egg, chopped

In a large bowl, combine potatoes, celery, and onion. In a small bowl, combine mayonnaise, sugar substitute, vinegar, mustard, parsley flakes, and black pepper. Add mayonnaise mixture to potato mixture. Mix well to combine. Fold in egg. Cover and refrigerate for at least 30 minutes. Gently stir again just before serving.

HINT: If you want the look and feel of egg without the cholesterol, toss out the yolk and dice the white.

Each serving equals:

HE: ¾ Bread • ½ Vegetable • ¼ Protein (limited) •
¼ Slider • 8 Optional Calories

105 Calories • 1 gm Fat • 3 gm Protein •
21 gm Carbohydrate • 474 mg Sodium •
28 mg Calcium • 2 gm Fiber

DIABETIC: 1½ Starch

Baked Potato Salad

Mmm, doesn't just the name of this dish get your taste buds excited? I combined the flavors of that popular restaurant appetizer, baked potato skins, then banished the fat without losing the mouth-watering taste we all love! Yum!　　◐　　Serves 4

2½ cups (12 ounces) cubed cooked potatoes

½ cup chopped celery

½ cup chopped onion

¾ cup (3 ounces) shredded Kraft reduced-fat Cheddar cheese☆

2 hard-boiled eggs, chopped

⅓ cup Kraft fat-free mayonnaise

2 tablespoons vinegar

⅛ teaspoon black pepper

Sugar substitute to equal 1 teaspoon sugar

1 teaspoon prepared mustard

Preheat oven to 350 degrees. Spray an 8-by-8-inch baking dish with butter-flavored cooking spray. In a large bowl, combine potatoes, celery, onion, half of Cheddar cheese, and eggs. In a small bowl, combine mayonnaise, vinegar, black pepper, sugar substitute, and mustard. Add mayonnaise mixture to potato mixture. Mix gently to combine. Spread mixture in prepared baking dish. Sprinkle remaining Cheddar cheese evenly over top. Bake for 30 minutes. Place baking dish on a wire rack and let set for 5 minutes. Divide into 4 servings.

HINT:　If you want the look and feel of eggs without the cholesterol, toss out the yolk and dice the whites.

Each serving equals:

HE: 1½ Protein (½ limited) • ¾ Bread •
½ Vegetable • 16 Optional Calories

166 Calories • 6 gm Fat • 10 gm Protein •
18 gm Carbohydrate • 573 mg Sodium •
170 mg Calcium • 2 gm Fiber

DIABETIC: 1½ Starch • 1 Meat

Luck of the Irish Pea Salad

Aren't peas one of nature's more perfect packages? So much goodness in one tiny bite! Here's a recipe that takes what's already downright delectable and makes it truly scrumptious! Those little bits of ham and cheese might start you singing.

☻ Serves 4 (½ cup)

> 2 cups (one 16-ounce can) tiny peas, rinsed and drained
> 1 (2.5-ounce) package Carl Buddig 90% lean ham, finely shredded
> ⅓ cup (1½ ounces) shredded Kraft reduced-fat Cheddar cheese
> ½ cup Kraft fat-free mayonnaise
> Sugar substitute to equal 1 tablespoon sugar
> 1 teaspoon lemon juice
> 1 teaspoon dried onion flakes
> ¼ teaspoon black pepper

In a medium bowl, combine peas, ham, and Cheddar cheese. In a small bowl, combine mayonnaise, sugar substitute, lemon juice, onion flakes, and black pepper. Add mayonnaise mixture to pea mixture. Mix gently to combine. Refrigerate for at least 30 minutes. Gently stir again just before serving.

Each serving equals:

HE: 1 Bread • 1 Protein • ¼ Slider •
2 Optional Calories

---

140 Calories • 4 gm Fat • 10 gm Protein •
16 gm Carbohydrate • 596 mg Sodium •
88 mg Calcium • 4 gm Fiber

DIABETIC: 1 Starch • 1 Meat

Smorgasbord Pea Salad

I love olives, and they have such an intense flavor, just a small amount goes a long way! They give this creamy pea salad some extra punch—and may even make you smile with satisfaction.

☻ Serves 4 (¾ cup)

2 cups frozen peas, thawed
¾ cup finely chopped celery
¼ cup finely chopped onion
¼ cup (1 ounce) sliced ripe olives
1 hard-boiled egg, chopped
⅓ cup Kraft fat-free mayonnaise
2 tablespoons skim milk
Sugar substitute to equal 1 tablespoon sugar
¼ teaspoon black pepper
1 teaspoon dried parsley flakes

In a large bowl, combine peas, celery, onion, olives, and egg. In a small bowl, combine mayonnaise, skim milk, sugar substitute, black pepper, and parsley flakes. Add mayonnaise mixture to pea mixture. Mix gently to combine. Cover and refrigerate for at least 30 minutes. Gently stir again just before serving.

HINTS: 1. Thaw peas by placing in a colander and rinsing under hot water for one minute.
2. If you want the look and feel of eggs without the cholesterol, toss out the yolk and dice the white.

Each serving equals:

HE: 1 Bread • 1 Vegetable • ¼ Protein (limited) •
¼ Fat • ¼ Slider • 3 Optional Calories

110 Calories • 2 gm Fat • 6 gm Protein •
17 gm Carbohydrate • 289 mg Sodium •
54 mg Calcium • 4 gm Fiber

DIABETIC: 1 Starch • ½ Fat

Lillian's Pasta-Garden Salad

Named for the lady in Rock Island, Illinois, who inspired it, this colorful and crunchy salad sparkles with all the glories of the garden! And the seashell macaroni just gives it that "by-the-ocean" vacation sensation, doesn't it? ☺ Serves 6 (1 cup)

2 cups cooked shell macaroni, rinsed and drained
¼ cup sliced green onion
2 tablespoons Hormel Bacon Bits
⅔ cup Kraft fat-free mayonnaise
1 tablespoon lemon juice
2 tablespoons grated Kraft fat-free Parmesan cheese
Sugar substitute to equal 2 teaspoons sugar
¼ teaspoon dried minced garlic
1 cup finely shredded fresh spinach
¾ cup chopped fresh cauliflower
¾ cup chopped fresh broccoli
¾ cup chopped fresh tomatoes

In a large bowl, combine macaroni, onion, and bacon bits. In a small bowl, combine mayonnaise, lemon juice, Parmesan cheese, sugar substitute, and garlic. Add mayonnaise mixture to macaroni mixture. Mix well to combine. Stir in spinach, cauliflower, broccoli, and tomatoes. Cover and refrigerate for at least 30 minutes. Gently stir again just before serving.

HINT: 1¾ cups uncooked macaroni usually cooks to about 2 cups.

Each serving equals:

HE: 1⅓ Vegetable • ⅔ Bread • ¼ Slider •
11 Optional Calories

---

117 Calories • 1 gm Fat • 4 gm Protein •
23 gm Carbohydrate • 367 mg Sodium •
24 mg Calcium • 2 gm Fiber

DIABETIC: 1 Vegetable • 1 Starch

Catalina Veggie Pasta Salad

Here's a lively luncheon entree or side dish that is truly luscious—
and takes just a few moments to stir up! It's important to let the flavors "cuddle up" before serving, so give it a half hour or more in the
fridge before serving it on pretty lettuce leaves.

☺ Serves 4 (¾ cup)

> 2 cups cold cooked rotini pasta, rinsed and drained
> 1 cup shredded carrots
> ½ cup finely chopped celery
> ¼ cup chopped green bell pepper
> ¼ cup chopped onion
> ¼ cup Kraft fat-free mayonnaise
> ⅓ cup Kraft Fat Free Catalina Dressing
> 1 tablespoon sweet pickle relish

In a large bowl, combine rotini pasta, carrots, celery, green
pepper, and onion. In a small bowl, combine mayonnaise, Catalina
dressing, and pickle relish. Add mayonnaise mixture to pasta mixture. Mix well to combine. Cover and refrigerate for at least 30 minutes. Gently stir again just before serving.

HINT: 1½ cups uncooked rotini pasta usually cooks to about 2
cups.

Each serving equals:

HE: 1 Bread • 1 Vegetable • ½ Slider •
4 Optional Calories

---

157 Calories • 1 gm Fat • 4 gm Protein •
33 gm Carbohydrate • 405 mg Sodium •
22 mg Calcium • 3 gm Fiber

DIABETIC: 2 Starch • ½ Vegetable

Mediterranean Macaroni Salad

They say the blue-green water of the Mediterranean isn't like anything else on earth, and while I haven't seen it myself, I bet it's true. Can you imagine how pleasant it would be to sit in a seaside cafe and dine like royalty on this appetizing salad? Now, be adventurous: five years ago, I didn't know what feta cheese was. Now it's on my top-ten list of favorite foods! ☺ Serves 4 (1⅓ cups)

2 cups cold cooked elbow macaroni, rinsed and drained
¼ cup (1 ounce) sliced ripe olives
1 cup chopped unpeeled cucumber
¾ cup chopped fresh tomatoes
¼ cup chopped red onion
¾ cup (3 ounces) crumbled feta cheese
½ cup Kraft Fat Free Italian Dressing
¼ cup Kraft fat-free mayonnaise
Sugar substitute to equal 2 teaspoons sugar

In a large bowl, combine macaroni, olives, cucumber, tomatoes, onion, and feta cheese. In a small bowl, combine Italian dressing, mayonnaise, and sugar substitute. Add dressing mixture to macaroni mixture. Mix well to combine. Cover and refrigerate for at least 30 minutes. Gently stir again just before serving.

HINT: 1⅓ cups uncooked elbow macaroni usually cooks to about 2 cups.

Each serving equals:

HE: 1½ Vegetable • 1 Bread • 1 Protein • ¼ Fat • 19 Optional Calories

202 Calories • 6 gm Fat • 7 gm Protein • 30 gm Carbohydrate • 755 mg Sodium • 124 mg Calcium • 2 gm Fiber

DIABETIC: 1½ Starch • 1 Meat • 1 Vegetable • ½ Fat

Seashell Tuna Salad

I think one of the fun things about making a pasta salad with shell macaroni is that once you've stirred all your ingredients together and you start to eat, you keep finding little bits of yummy flavors hidden inside each shell! It makes each forkful a little extra-special.

◐ Serves 4 (1 cup)

1½ cups cold cooked seashell macaroni, rinsed and drained
½ cup frozen peas, thawed
1 cup chopped celery
1 (6-ounce) can white tuna, packed in water, drained and flaked
½ cup Kraft fat-free mayonnaise
2 teaspoons white vinegar
Sugar substitute to equal 2 teaspoons sugar
1 teaspoon prepared mustard
1 tablespoon dried parsley flakes
1 teaspoon dried onion flakes

In a large bowl, combine macaroni, peas, celery, and tuna. In a small bowl, combine mayonnaise, vinegar, sugar substitute, mustard, parsley flakes, and onion flakes. Add mayonnaise mixture to macaroni mixture. Mix gently to combine. Cover and refrigerate for at least 1 hour. Gently stir again just before serving.

HINTS: 1. 1 cup uncooked seashell macaroni usually cooks to about 1½ cups.
2. Thaw peas by placing in a colander and rinsing under hot water for one minute.

Each serving equals:

HE: 1 Bread • ¾ Protein • ½ Vegetable • ¼ Slider • 1 Optional Calorie

161 Calories • 1 gm Fat • 15 gm Protein • 23 gm Carbohydrate • 400 mg Sodium • 39 mg Calcium • 2 gm Fiber

DIABETIC: 1½ Starch • 1½ Meat

Curried Turkey and Peanut Salad

If you haven't cooked with curry, you may wonder if adding this Indian spice to a dish will make it too hot. It really won't! In this dish, the curry, along with other spices, adds more of a richness of flavor than actual heat. If you've always wanted to experience the exotic without leaving home, give this salad a try.

● Serves 4 (¾ cup)

> ½ cup Kraft fat-free mayonnaise
> 2 tablespoons Peter Pan reduced-fat chunky peanut butter
> 2 tablespoons Land O Lakes no-fat sour cream
> 1 cup (one 8-ounce can) pineapple tidbits, packed in fruit juice, drained, and 2 tablespoons liquid reserved
> ½ teaspoon curry powder
> ¼ teaspoon turmeric
> ¼ teaspoon ground ginger
> 1½ cups (8 ounces) diced cooked turkey breast
> ¼ cup (1 ounce) chopped dry-roasted peanuts
> 1 cup chopped celery

In a large bowl, combine mayonnaise, peanut butter, sour cream, reserved pineapple liquid, curry powder, turmeric, and ginger. Add turkey, pineapple, peanuts, and celery. Mix well to combine. Cover and refrigerate for at least 30 minutes. Gently stir again just before serving. Good served over lettuce or stuffed in pita halves.

HINTS: 1. If you can't find tidbits, use chunk pineapple and coarsely chop.
2. If you don't have leftovers, purchase a chunk of cooked turkey breast from your local deli.

Each serving equals:

HE: 2¾ Protein • 1 Fat • ½ Fruit • ½ Vegetable • ¼ Slider • 8 Optional Calories

219 Calories • 7 gm Fat • 18 gm Protein • 21 gm Carbohydrate • 319 mg Sodium • 44 mg Calcium • 1 gm Fiber

DIABETIC: 3 Meat • 1 Fat • ½ Fruit • ½ Starch

Honey Mustard
Chicken Pasta Salad

Cliff isn't much of a pasta salad fan, but he liked this one quite a bit, probably because of the green beans and the honey mustard dressing. This cool salad is terrific on those steamy summer days when you're hungry and can't stand the heat!

○ Serves 4 (1 full cup)

2 cups cold cooked rotini pasta, rinsed and drained
1½ cups (8 ounces) diced cooked chicken breast
2 cups (one 16-ounce can) cut green beans, rinsed and drained
½ cup Kraft Fat Free Honey Mustard Dressing
¼ cup Kraft fat-free mayonnaise
1 teaspoon dried parsley flakes
¼ teaspoon black pepper

In a large bowl, combine rotini pasta, chicken, and green beans. In a small bowl, combine Honey Mustard dressing, mayonnaise, parsley flakes, and black pepper. Add dressing mixture to pasta mixture. Mix well to combine. Cover and refrigerate for at least 30 minutes. Gently stir again just before serving.

HINTS: 1. 1½ cups uncooked rotini pasta usually cooks to about 2 cups.
2. If you don't have leftovers, purchase a chunk of cooked chicken breast from your local deli.

Each serving equals:

HE: 2 Protein • 1 Bread • 1 Vegetable • ½ Slider • 10 Optional Calories

255 Calories • 3 gm Fat • 22 gm Protein • 35 gm Carbohydrate • 341 mg Sodium • 40 mg Calcium • 2 gm Fiber

DIABETIC: 2 Meat • 2 Starch • 1 Vegetable

Picnic Macaroni Salad

Whether it's the Fourth of July or just a meal with friends by the lake, you'll find this lively macaroni salad packs plenty of culinary fireworks! As with any salad containing mayonnaise, make sure to keep it cold until it's time to eat.   ☽   Serves 6 (1 full cup)

3 cups cold cooked elbow macaroni, rinsed and drained
¾ cup (3 ounces) shredded Kraft reduced-fat Cheddar cheese
1 full cup (6 ounces) diced Dubuque 97% fat-free ham or any
*   extra-lean ham*
¼ cup chopped onion
¾ cup chopped celery
1 cup chopped fresh tomatoes
¼ cup sweet pickle relish
½ cup Kraft fat-free mayonnaise
1 teaspoon prepared mustard
¼ teaspoon black pepper

In a large bowl, combine macaroni, Cheddar cheese, ham, onion, celery, and tomatoes. In a small bowl, combine pickle relish, mayonnaise, mustard, and black pepper. Add mayonnaise mixture to macaroni mixture. Mix well to combine. Cover and refrigerate for at least 30 minutes. Gently stir again just before serving.

HINT: 2½ cups uncooked macaroni usually cooks to about 3 cups.

Each serving equals:

HE: 1⅓ Protein • 1 Bread • ⅔ Vegetable • ¼ Slider • 1 Optional Calorie

204 Calories • 4 gm Fat • 12 gm Protein • 30 gm Carbohydrate • 632 mg Sodium • 110 mg Calcium • 2 gm Fiber

DIABETIC: 1½ Starch • 1 Meat • 1 Vegetable

Letts Picnic Pasta Salad

I created this mustardy pasta salad at the request of a Healthy Exchanges fan from Letts, Iowa, when I went there to give a talk. Don't you think the hot dogs are a festive touch for a picnic salad, but served in this unexpected way? ☻ Serves 4 (1 cup)

> 8 ounces Healthy Choice 97% fat-free frankfurters, cooked,
>   cooled, and diced
> 1 cup chopped celery
> 2 cups cold cooked rotini pasta, rinsed and drained
> ½ cup Kraft fat-free mayonnaise
> 1 tablespoon Dijon mustard
> 1 tablespoon dried parsley flakes
> Sugar substitute to equal 2 teaspoons sugar

In a large bowl, combine frankfurters, celery, and rotini pasta. In a small bowl, combine mayonnaise, mustard, parsley flakes, and sugar substitute. Add mayonnaise mixture to frankfurter mixture. Mix well to combine. Cover and refrigerate for at least 30 minutes. Gently stir again just before serving.

HINTS: 1. 1½ cups uncooked rotini pasta usually cooks to about 2 cups.
         2. 1 full cup (6 ounces) diced 97% fat-free ham may be substituted for frankfurters.

Each serving equals:

HE: 1⅓ Protein • 1 Bread • ½ Vegetable • ¼ Slider • 1 Optional Calorie

186 Calories • 2 gm Fat • 11 gm Protein •
31 gm Carbohydrate • 953 mg Sodium •
22 mg Calcium • 1 gm Fiber

DIABETIC: 2 Starch • 1½ Meat

Sweet Salads

Fresh Fruit Cup

Never thought of pouring ginger ale over fresh fruit to give it an extra zing? Oh, try it—and you may never want to eat your berries again without bubbles!   ☻   Serves 2

> 1 cup sliced fresh strawberries
> ½ cup (3 ounces) sliced green seedless grapes
> ¾ cup fresh blueberries
> ¼ cup diet ginger ale

In a medium bowl, combine strawberries, grapes, and blueberries. Evenly divide fruit mixture between 2 parfait dishes. Pour 2 tablespoons diet ginger ale over each. Refrigerate for at least 30 minutes.

Each serving equals:

HE: 1½ Fruit

80 Calories • 0 gm Fat • 1 gm Protein • 19 gm Carbohydrate • 10 mg Sodium • 18 mg Calcium • 3 gm Fiber

DIABETIC: 1½ Fruit

Deliteful Mandarin Orange Salad

Here's a fast and luscious blend that stirs up in the most beautiful shade of pale orange! It's a sort of cousin to the popular dish called ambrosia, which also celebrates the sweetness of fruit by mixing in marshmallows and coconut. Why not try it at your next special occasion? It goes just great with ham, turkey, or roast beef.

❂ Serves 6 (⅔ cup)

> ¾ cup Yoplait plain fat-free yogurt
> ⅓ cup Carnation Nonfat Dry Milk Powder
> 1 (4-serving) package JELL-O sugar-free orange gelatin
> ¾ cup Cool Whip Free
> 1 teaspoon coconut extract
> 2 cups (two 11-ounce cans) mandarin oranges, rinsed and
>   drained
> ½ cup (½ ounce) miniature marshmallows
> 2 tablespoons flaked coconut

In a medium bowl, combine yogurt and dry milk powder. Add dry gelatin. Mix well to combine. Fold in Cool Whip Free and coconut extract. Add mandarin oranges, marshmallows, and coconut. Mix gently to combine. Cover and refrigerate for at least 15 minutes. Gently stir again just before serving.

Each serving equals:

HE: ⅔ Fruit • ⅓ Skim Milk • ½ Slider

96 Calories • 0 gm Fat • 4 gm Protein •
20 gm Carbohydrate • 93 mg Sodium •
112 mg Calcium • 0 gm Fiber

DIABETIC: 1 Starch/Carbohydrate

Holiday Sparkle Salad

I think layered salads are especially festive around Christmas or Thanksgiving, especially when they're sweet and colorful like this one! The nuts, apples, and celery provide a really satisfying crunch—but the topping is so creamy, the contrast is perfect.   ☻   Serves 8

1 (4-serving) package JELL-O sugar-free raspberry gelatin
¾ cup boiling water
1 cup Ocean Spray reduced-calorie cranberry juice cocktail
1½ cups (3 small) cored, unpeeled, and diced Red Delicious
    apples
1 cup chopped celery
2 tablespoons (½ ounce) chopped pecans
1 (4-serving) package JELL-O sugar-free lemon gelatin
1 cup Diet Mountain Dew
1 cup Cool Whip Free
½ cup Kraft fat-free mayonnaise

In a large bowl, combine dry raspberry gelatin and boiling water. Mix well to dissolve gelatin. Stir in cranberry juice cocktail. Refrigerate for 15 minutes. Stir in apples, celery, and pecans. Pour mixture into an 8-by-8-inch dish. Refrigerate while preparing topping. Meanwhile, in a medium saucepan, combine dry lemon gelatin and Diet Mountain Dew. Bring mixture to a boil. Remove from heat. Refrigerate for 30 minutes. Stir in Cool Whip Free and mayonnaise. Spread topping mixture evenly over partially set raspberry gelatin mixture. Refrigerate until firm, about 3 hours. Cut into 8 servings.

Each serving equals:

HE: ½ Fruit • ¼ Vegetable • ¼ Fat • ¼ Slider • 16 Optional Calories

61 Calories • 1 gm Fat • 1 gm Protein •
12 gm Carbohydrate • 210 mg Sodium •
8 mg Calcium • 1 gm Fiber

DIABETIC: 1 Fruit *or* 1 Starch/Carbohydrate

Pineapple Waldorf Salad

One of the best pieces of recipe-creating advice I can share—don't be afraid to "monkey" with the classics! I took the original Waldorf salad blend, then mixed in a little tropical surprise for a great new taste. Maybe you've got an idea how to make another classic dish your own. . . .   ☮   Serves 6 (1 cup)

2 cups (4 small) cored, unpeeled, and diced Red Delicious apples
1 cup diced celery
¼ cup raisins
¼ cup (1 ounce) chopped walnuts
⅓ cup Kraft fat-free mayonnaise
⅔ cup Cool Whip Free
1 cup (one 8-ounce can) crushed pineapple, packed in fruit juice, drained
1 teaspoon lemon juice

In a large bowl, combine apples, celery, raisins, and walnuts. In a medium bowl, combine mayonnaise, Cool Whip Free, pineapple, and lemon juice. Add mayonnaise mixture to apple mixture. Mix well to combine. Cover and refrigerate for at least 30 minutes. Gently stir again just before serving.

HINT: To plump up raisins without "cooking," place in a glass measuring cup and microwave on HIGH for 20 seconds.

Each serving equals:

HE: 1⅓ Fruit • ⅓ Vegetable • ⅓ Fat • ¼ Slider • 16 Optional Calories

127 Calories • 3 gm Fat • 1 gm Protein • 24 gm Carbohydrate • 138 mg Sodium • 24 mg Calcium • 2 gm Fiber

DIABETIC: 1 Fruit • ½ Starch • ½ Fat

Festive Cranberry Salad

You could almost build your next party around this beautiful creation, it's such an ideal centerpiece! In fact, instead of serving it in six individual dishes, you might choose to present it in a cut glass bowl that once belonged to your mother or grandmother. Now, doesn't that just make you want to celebrate?

♥ Serves 6

> 1 (4-serving) package JELL-O sugar-free cranberry or raspberry gelatin
>
> 1 (4-serving) package JELL-O sugar-free vanilla cook-and-serve pudding mix
>
> 1 cup (one 8-ounce can) crushed pineapple, packed in fruit juice, undrained
>
> ⅓ cup water
>
> 2 cups fresh or frozen cranberries
>
> ¾ cup Yoplait plain fat-free yogurt
>
> ⅓ cup Carnation Nonfat Dry Milk Powder
>
> Sugar substitute to equal 2 tablespoons sugar
>
> 1 teaspoon vanilla extract
>
> ½ cup Cool Whip Free
>
> 1 cup (1 medium) diced banana

In a medium saucepan, combine dry gelatin and dry pudding mix. Stir in undrained pineapple, water, and cranberries. Cook over medium heat until mixture starts to boil and cranberries soften, stirring constantly. Remove from heat. Place saucepan on a wire rack and allow to cool for 1 hour. In a medium bowl, combine yogurt and dry milk powder. Stir in sugar substitute and vanilla extract. Add cooled cranberry mixture to yogurt mixture. Mix well to combine. Fold in Cool Whip Free and banana. Spoon mixture into 6 individual serving dishes. Refrigerate for at least 30 minutes.

HINT: To prevent banana from turning brown, mix with 1 teaspoon lemon juice or sprinkle with Fruit Fresh.

Each serving equals:

HE: 1 Fruit • ⅓ Skim Milk • ¼ Slider •
15 Optional Calories

124 Calories • 0 gm Fat • 4 gm Protein •
27 gm Carbohydrate • 159 mg Sodium •
112 mg Calcium • 2 gm Fiber

DIABETIC: 1 Fruit • ½ Starch

Jean's Creamy Lemon Waldorf Salad

Here's another way to take a flavor you enjoy (for me, it's lemon, lemon, lemon) and mingle it with familiar ingredients to make something delectably new and fun! This dish is creamy and rich, a lovely choice for a luncheon or card party.

☻ Serves 6 (⅔ cup)

> 1 (4-serving) package JELL-O sugar-free instant vanilla pudding mix
> 1 (4-serving) package JELL-O sugar-free lemon gelatin
> ⅔ cup Carnation Nonfat Dry Milk Powder
> 1⅓ cups water
> ¾ cup Cool Whip Free
> ¾ cup finely chopped celery
> 2 cups (4 small) cored, unpeeled, and chopped Red Delicious apples
> ¼ cup (1 ounce) chopped walnuts

In a large bowl, combine dry pudding mix, dry gelatin, dry milk powder, and water. Mix well using a wire whisk. Blend in Cool Whip Free. Add celery, apples, and walnuts. Mix gently to combine. Cover and refrigerate for at least 30 minutes. Gently stir again just before serving.

Each serving equals:

HE: ⅔ Fruit • ⅓ Skim Milk • ⅓ Fat • ¼ Vegetable • ½ Slider • 13 Optional Calories

---

119 Calories • 3 gm Fat • 4 gm Protein • 19 gm Carbohydrate • 316 mg Sodium • 105 mg Calcium • 1 gm Fiber

---

DIABETIC: 1 Fruit • ½ Starch • ½ Fat

Hawaiian Waldorf Salad

Maybe it's those special sea winds or the sun that shines so bright in the tropics, but pineapple always seems to have such a heavenly flavor! Stirred together with grapes and apples, combined with the crunch of celery and nuts, this dish will urge your taste buds to get you on a plane to Hawaii!   ☾   Serves 6 (⅔ cup)

> 2 cups (4 small) cored, unpeeled, and chopped Red Delicious
>   apples
> 1 cup chopped celery
> 1 cup (6 ounces) sliced green seedless grapes
> 1 cup (one 8-ounce can) pineapple tidbits, packed in fruit juice,
>   drained, and 2 tablespoons liquid reserved
> 2 tablespoons (½ ounce) chopped pecans
> ¼ cup Kraft fat-free mayonnaise

In a medium bowl, combine apples, celery, grapes, pineapple, and pecans. In a small bowl, combine mayonnaise and 2 tablespoons reserved pineapple liquid. Add mayonnaise mixture to apple mixture. Mix gently to combine. Cover and refrigerate for at least 30 minutes. Gently stir again just before serving.

HINT: If you can't find tidbits, use chunk pineapple and coarsely chop.

Each serving equals:

HE: 1 Fruit • ⅓ Vegetable • ⅓ Fat •
7 Optional Calories

---

98 Calories • 2 gm Fat • 0 gm Protein •
20 gm Carbohydrate • 105 mg Sodium •
20 mg Calcium • 2 gm Fiber

DIABETIC: 1 Fruit • ½ Fat

Fruited Party Salad

Don't let the name fool you—this pretty dish isn't only for special occasions, although it does take a bit more time to prepare because it's layered. And because it uses fruits that are available most all year round, you can "party" anytime at all!   ☺   Serves 8

2 (4-serving) packages JELL-O sugar-free lemon gelatin

1½ cups boiling water

1½ cups Diet Mountain Dew

1 cup (6 ounces) halved white seedless grapes

1 cup (2 small) cored, unpeeled, and chopped Red Delicious apples

1 cup (one 11-ounce can) mandarin oranges, rinsed and drained

¾ cup Yoplait plain fat-free yogurt

⅓ cup Carnation Nonfat Dry Milk Powder

Sugar substitute to equal ¼ cup sugar

1 teaspoon vanilla extract

1 cup Cool Whip Free

1 cup (one 8-ounce can) crushed pineapple, packed in fruit juice, drained

In a large bowl, combine dry gelatin and boiling water. Mix well to dissolve gelatin. Stir in Diet Mountain Dew. Allow to cool until foam subsides. Add grapes, apples, and oranges. Mix gently to combine. Pour mixture into an 8-by-8-inch dish. Refrigerate until firm, about 3 hours. In a medium bowl, combine yogurt and dry milk powder. Add sugar substitute, vanilla extract, and Cool Whip Free. Mix gently to combine. Fold in pineapple. Spread topping mixture evenly over set gelatin. Refrigerate for at least 30 minutes. Cut into 8 servings.

Each serving equals:

HE: 1 Fruit • ¼ Skim Milk • ¼ Slider •
7 Optional Calories

100 Calories • 0 gm Fat • 4 gm Protein •
21 gm Carbohydrate • 98 mg Sodium •
88 mg Calcium • 1 gm Fiber

DIABETIC: 1 Fruit • ½ Starch

Grandma's Apple Salad

Sometimes, something sweet on the side of a plate just makes a meal complete. This fast and fruity salad is perfect for those times when you've got no time—but you still want to nurture your family and yourself. The marshmallows make it fun, and the raisins are so full of old-fashioned goodness, they remind me of baking with Grandma. (Remember her good advice about an apple a day keeping the doctor away, too!)　　　❍　　　Serves 6 (⅔ cup)

> 3 cups (6 small) cored, unpeeled, and diced Red Delicious apples
> ¼ cup raisins
> 1 cup (one 8-ounce can) crushed pineapple, packed in fruit juice, drained, and 2 tablespoons liquid reserved
> ½ cup (1 ounce) miniature marshmallows
> ½ cup Kraft fat-free mayonnaise
> Sugar substitute to equal 2 tablespoons sugar

In a medium bowl, combine apples, raisins, pineapple, and marshmallows. In a small bowl, combine mayonnaise, sugar substitute, and reserved pineapple liquid. Add mayonnaise mixture to apple mixture. Mix gently to combine. Cover and refrigerate for at least 30 minutes. Gently stir again just before serving.

HINT:　To plump up raisins without "cooking," place in a glass measuring cup and microwave on HIGH for 20 seconds.

Each serving equals:

HE: 1⅓ Fruit • ¼ Slider • 4 Optional Calories

104 Calories • 0 gm Fat • 0 gm Protein •
26 gm Carbohydrate • 176 mg Sodium •
13 mg Calcium • 2 gm Fiber

DIABETIC: 1½ Fruit *or* 1 Fruit • ½ Starch/Carbohydrate

Lemon Fruit Fluff Salad

The tradition of sweet salads was born in the Midwest, but I've done all I can to spread the word! This one is so easy, even kids and teens can stir it up in no time at all. (It was a big hit with my grandsons, Zach and Josh!) Even men who think they don't like "fluff" will love this sensational lemon treat. ☺ Serves 6 (⅔ cup)

1 (4-serving) package JELL-O sugar-free instant vanilla pudding mix

1 (4-serving) package JELL-O sugar-free lemon gelatin

⅔ cup Carnation Nonfat Dry Milk Powder

1 cup (one 8-ounce can) fruit cocktail, packed in fruit juice, drained, and ¼ cup liquid reserved

¾ cup water

¾ cup Cool Whip Free

1 cup (one 8-ounce can) crushed pineapple, packed in fruit juice, undrained

1 cup (1 medium) diced banana

½ cup (1 ounce) miniature marshmallows

2 tablespoons (½ ounce) chopped pecans

In a large bowl, combine dry pudding mix, dry gelatin, and dry milk powder. Add reserved fruit cocktail liquid and water. Mix well using a wire whisk. Blend in Cool Whip Free. Add pineapple, banana, fruit cocktail, marshmallows, and pecans. Mix gently to combine. Cover and refrigerate for at least 30 minutes. Gently stir again just before serving.

HINT: To prevent banana from turning brown, mix with 1 teaspoon lemon juice or sprinkle with Fruit Fresh.

Each serving equals:

HE: 1 Fruit • ⅓ Skim Milk • ⅓ Fat • ½ Slider • 11 Optional Calories

157 Calories • 1 gm Fat • 4 gm Protein • 33 gm Carbohydrate • 306 mg Sodium • 104 mg Calcium • 1 gm Fiber

DIABETIC: 1 Fruit • 1 Starch • ½ Fat

Summer Banana Salad

This pretty seasonal dish is at its best when the blueberries are so ripe and plump, they almost pop! And between the pudding and the fruit itself, you'll really taste the richness of the banana flavor!

○ Serves 8 (¾ cup)

> 1 (4-serving) package JELL-O sugar-free instant banana cream pudding mix
> ⅓ cup Carnation Nonfat Dry Milk Powder
> ¾ cup Yoplait plain fat-free yogurt
> 1 cup (one 8-ounce can) crushed pineapple, packed in fruit juice, undrained
> ¾ cup water
> ¾ cup Cool Whip Free
> 2 cups (2 medium) diced bananas
> 1½ cups fresh blueberries

In a medium bowl, combine dry pudding mix and dry milk powder. Add yogurt, undrained pineapple, and water. Mix well using a wire whisk. Blend in Cool Whip Free. Add bananas and blueberries. Mix gently to combine. Cover and refrigerate for at least 1 hour. Gently stir again just before serving.

HINT: To prevent bananas from turning brown, mix with 1 teaspoon lemon juice or sprinkle with Fruit Fresh.

Each serving equals:

HE: 1 Fruit • ¼ Skim Milk • ¼ Slider •
8 Optional Calories

---

116 Calories • 0 gm Fat • 3 gm Protein •
26 gm Carbohydrate • 207 mg Sodium •
85 mg Calcium • 2 gm Fiber

DIABETIC: 1 Fruit • ½ Starch

Peach Salad

Aren't peaches just a heavenly fruit, even in their canned form? This recipe celebrates that sweet flavor in a concoction that's really rich and creamy too! This would be pretty served as part of a brunch.

● Serves 8

2 cups (one 16-ounce can) sliced peaches, packed in fruit juice, drained

1 (4-serving) package JELL-O sugar-free lemon gelatin

1 cup (one 8-ounce can) crushed pineapple, packed in fruit juice, undrained

1 (8-ounce) package Philadelphia fat-free cream cheese

1 (4-serving) package JELL-O sugar-free instant vanilla pudding mix

2 cups skim milk

1 cup Cool Whip Free

Chop peaches and drain thoroughly. Set aside. In a medium saucepan, combine dry gelatin and undrained pineapple. Cook over medium heat until mixture thickens and starts to boil, stirring constantly. Remove from heat. Place saucepan on a wire rack and allow to cool for 20 minutes. In a large bowl, stir cream cheese with a spoon until soft. Add dry pudding mix and skim milk. Mix well using a wire whisk. Blend in Cool Whip Free, drained peaches, and cooled pineapple mixture. Pour mixture into a 9-by-13-inch pan. Refrigerate until firm, about 3 hours. Cut into 8 servings.

Each serving equals:

HE: ¾ Fruit • ½ Protein • ¼ Skim Milk • ¼ Slider • 13 Optional Calories

---

116 Calories • 0 gm Fat • 7 gm Protein • 22 gm Carbohydrate • 294 mg Sodium • 83 mg Calcium • 1 gm Fiber

---

DIABETIC: 1 Fruit • ½ Meat • ½ Starch

Peach Melba Gelatin Salad

The traditional peach melba dish combines peaches and raspberries, but somehow adding the mini-marshmallows turns an ordinary dish into one your family will cheer. This could also be poured into a mold for a special occasion.　　**◐**　　Serves 6

1 (4-serving) package JELL-O sugar-free raspberry gelatin
¾ cup boiling water
2 cups (one 16-ounce can) sliced peaches, packed in fruit juice,
　　　drained, and ¼ cup liquid reserved
1½ cups frozen unsweetened red raspberries
½ cup (1 ounce) miniature marshmallows

In a large bowl, combine dry gelatin and boiling water. Mix well to dissolve gelatin. Add reserved peach liquid and frozen raspberries. Mix gently to combine, being careful not to crush raspberries. Refrigerate for 15 minutes. Coarsely chop peaches. Gently stir peaches and marshmallows into gelatin mixture. Pour mixture into an 8-by-8-inch dish. Refrigerate until firm, about 3 hours. Cut into 6 servings.

Each serving equals:

HE: 1 Fruit • 15 Optional Calories

68 Calories • 0 gm Fat • 1 gm Protein •
16 gm Carbohydrate • 41 mg Sodium •
12 mg Calcium • 2 gm Fiber

DIABETIC: 1 Fruit

Upstate Cherry Salad

My friend Barbara gave me the idea for this salad when she described a favorite ice cream flavor that combined bing cherries and chunks of chocolate. She declared this dish was a tasty and healthy way to enjoy the flavors she loves!

◐ Serves 6 (⅔ cup)

> 1 (4-serving) package JELL-O sugar-free instant vanilla pudding mix
> ⅔ cup Carnation Nonfat Dry Milk Powder
> 1¼ cups water
> 1 teaspoon vanilla extract
> ¾ cup Yoplait plain fat-free yogurt
> ¾ cup Cool Whip Free
> ¼ cup (1 ounce) mini chocolate chips
> 2 cups (12 ounces) frozen unsweetened pitted bing or sweet cherries, thawed and drained

In a large bowl, combine dry pudding mix, dry milk powder, and water. Mix well using a wire whisk. Blend in vanilla extract, yogurt, and Cool Whip Free. Add chocolate chips and bing cherries. Mix gently to combine. Cover and refrigerate for at least 30 minutes. Gently stir again just before serving.

HINT: If you can't find frozen sweet cherries, buy the canned version packed in heavy syrup, place in a colander, and rinse well under cold water.

Each serving equals:

HE: ⅔ Fruit • ½ Skim Milk • ¾ Slider •
2 Optional Calories

142 Calories • 2 gm Fat • 5 gm Protein •
26 gm Carbohydrate • 288 mg Sodium •
158 mg Calcium • 1 gm Fiber

DIABETIC: 1 Fruit • ½ Skim Milk • ½ Fat

Grandma's Easter Salad

When the family is gathered for Easter, there's no better time to serve this creamy fruited salad! The nuts and celery give it crunch, and the cheese provides an intriguing, savory touch that makes it special.   ◑   Serves 6 (⅔ cup)

   1 cup chopped celery
   ½ cup (1 ounce) miniature marshmallows
   3 tablespoons (¾ ounce) chopped pecans
   ¾ cup (3 ounces) shredded Kraft reduced-fat Cheddar cheese
   1 cup (one 8-ounce can) pineapple chunks, packed in fruit juice, drained, and ⅓ cup liquid reserved
   1 (4-serving) package JELL-O sugar-free vanilla cook-and-serve pudding mix
   ⅔ cup Carnation Nonfat Dry Milk Powder
   1 cup (one 8-ounce can) crushed pineapple, packed in fruit juice, undrained
   ⅔ cup water
   1 teaspoon vanilla extract
   ¾ cup Cool Whip Free

In a large bowl, combine celery, marshmallows, pecans, Cheddar cheese, and pineapple chunks. Cover and refrigerate. Meanwhile, in a medium saucepan, combine dry pudding mix, dry milk powder, undrained crushed pineapple, reserved pineapple liquid, and water. Cook over medium heat until mixture thickens and starts to boil, stirring constantly. Remove from heat. Stir in vanilla extract. Place saucepan on a wire rack and allow to cool for 20 minutes. Blend in Cool Whip Free. Add pudding mixture to celery mixture. Mix gently to combine. Cover and refrigerate for at least 2 hours. Gently stir again just before serving.

Each serving equals:

HE: ⅔ Protein • ⅔ Fruit • ½ Fat • ⅓ Vegetable •
⅓ Skim Milk • ½ Slider • 2 Optional Calories

157 Calories • 5 gm Fat • 7 gm Protein •
21 gm Carbohydrate • 264 mg Sodium •
215 mg Calcium • 1 gm Fiber

DIABETIC: 1 Fruit • ½ Meat • ½ Fat • ½ Starch

Fruit Pasta Salad

If you've never imagined a pasta salad served with fruit, go on—live a little! It's unusual but surprisingly good, especially if you (like Cliff) really adore fruit cocktail.   ❂   Serves 6 (⅔ cup)

> 2 cups cold cooked small shell macaroni, rinsed and drained
> 2 cups (one 16-ounce can) fruit cocktail, packed in fruit juice, drained
> 1 cup (1 medium) sliced banana
> ½ cup Cool Whip Free
> ¼ teaspoon apple pie spice

In a medium bowl, combine macaroni, fruit cocktail, and banana. Add Cool Whip Free and apple pie spice. Cover and refrigerate for at least 30 minutes. Gently stir again just before serving.

HINTS: 1. 1⅓ cups uncooked small shell macaroni usually cooks to about 2 cups.
   2. To prevent banana from turning brown, mix with 1 teaspoon lemon juice or sprinkle with Fruit Fresh.

Each serving equals:

HE: 1 Fruit • ⅔ Bread • 11 Optional Calories

137 Calories • 1 gm Fat • 3 gm Protein •
29 gm Carbohydrate • 225 mg Sodium •
18 mg Calcium • 2 gm Fiber

DIABETIC: 1 Fruit • 1 Starch

Main Dishes

HINT: Some of these recipes call for cooked chicken or turkey. If you don't have leftovers, do what I do—purchase a chunk of cooked meat from your local deli.

Three Cheese Strata

If one cheese is good, and two even better, why not go culinarily wild and enjoy three scrumptious (but low-fat or reduced-fat) cheeses? Take note: This wonderful baked bread and cheese combo needs to rest for at least an hour before baking—and can be prepared up to 24 hours in advance.   ☻   Serves 8

> *12 slices reduced-calorie Italian bread, cut into 1-inch cubes*
> *1 (10¾-ounce) can Healthy Request Cream of Mushroom Soup*
> *⅔ cup Carnation Nonfat Dry Milk Powder*
> *1½ cups water*
> *4 eggs, beaten, or equivalent in egg substitute*
> *¼ cup (¾ ounce) grated Kraft fat-free Parmesan cheese*
> *1½ cups (6 ounces) shredded Kraft reduced-fat Cheddar cheese*
> *7 (¾-ounce) slices Kraft reduced-fat Swiss cheese, shredded*

Spray a 9-by-13-inch baking dish with butter-flavored cooking spray. Evenly arrange bread cubes in prepared baking dish. In a large bowl, combine mushroom soup, dry milk powder, water, and eggs. Stir in Parmesan cheese, Cheddar cheese, and Swiss cheese. Pour soup mixture evenly over bread. Cover and refrigerate for at least 1 hour or up to 24 hours. Uncover and bake at 350 degrees for 45 minutes or until a knife inserted near center comes out clean. Place baking dish on a wire rack and let set for 5 minutes. Cut into 8 servings.

Each serving equals:

HE: 2½ Protein (½ limited) • ¾ Bread •
¼ Skim Milk • ¼ Slider • 1 Optional Calorie

---

227 Calories • 7 gm Fat • 22 gm Protein •
19 gm Carbohydrate • 603 mg Sodium •
272 mg Calcium • 0 gm Fiber

DIABETIC: 2 Meat • 1½ Starch

Veggie Mac and Cheese

Macaroni and cheese is always a man-pleasing and kid-pleasing entree, but if you're trying to get more veggies into your family's menu, here's a sly but savory way to do it! Again, I've "tucked" three different cheeses into this dish, which gives it an exceptionally delicious flavor. ☻ Serves 4

> 1 (10¾-ounce) can Healthy Request Cream of Mushroom Soup
> ⅓ cup Carnation Nonfat Dry Milk Powder
> ½ cup water
> ¼ cup (¾ ounce) grated Kraft fat-free Parmesan cheese
> ¾ cup (3 ounces) shredded Kraft reduced-fat Cheddar cheese
> ¾ cup (3 ounces) shredded Kraft reduced-fat mozzarella
>   cheese
> 2 cups hot cooked elbow macaroni, rinsed and drained
> 1 teaspoon dried parsley flakes
> ⅛ teaspoon black pepper
> 1 cup (one 8-ounce can) cut green beans, rinsed and drained
> 1 cup (one 8-ounce can) sliced carrots, rinsed and drained

Preheat oven to 350 degrees. Spray an 8-by-8-inch baking dish with butter-flavored cooking spray. In a large skillet, combine mushroom soup, dry milk powder, water, and Parmesan cheese. Stir in Cheddar and mozzarella cheese. Cook over medium heat until cheeses melt, stirring often. Add macaroni, parsley flakes, and black pepper. Mix well to combine. Stir in green beans and carrots. Spread mixture evenly into prepared baking dish. Bake for 30 minutes. Place baking dish on a wire rack and let set for 5 minutes. Divide into 4 servings.

HINT: 1⅓ cups uncooked elbow macaroni usually cooks to about 2 cups.

Each serving equals:

HE: 2¼ Protein • 1 Bread • 1 Vegetable •
¼ Skim Milk • ½ Slider • 1 Optional Calorie

296 Calories • 8 gm Fat • 21 gm Protein •
35 gm Carbohydrate • 745 mg Sodium •
421 mg Calcium • 3 gm Fiber

DIABETIC: 2 Meat • 2 Starch • 1 Vegetable

Tuscan White Bean Pizza

Wherever you look, someone's invented a new way to serve pizza—besides topped with cheese and pepperoni! Here's a variation that delivers healthy protein in the form of beans, coupled with lots of fresh veggies, for a meal that's good-tasting and good for you too.

◑ Serves 8

> 1 (8-ounce) can Pillsbury Reduced Fat Crescent Rolls
> ¼ cup Kraft Fat Free Italian Dressing
> ¼ cup (¾ ounce) grated Kraft fat-free Parmesan cheese
> 2 tablespoons chopped fresh parsley or 2 teaspoons dried parsley flakes
> 1½ cups peeled and chopped fresh tomatoes
> ¼ cup chopped onion
> ¼ cup chopped green bell pepper
> 10 ounces (one 16-ounce can) great northern beans, rinsed and drained
> 1½ cups (6 ounces) shredded Kraft reduced-fat mozzarella cheese

Preheat oven to 415 degrees. Spray a 12-inch pizza pan with olive oil–flavored cooking spray. Separate rolls into 8 triangles. Gently press dough to cover bottom of pan, being sure to seal perforations. Bake for 7 minutes. Meanwhile, in a large bowl, combine Italian dressing, Parmesan cheese, and parsley. Add tomatoes, onion, green pepper, and great northern beans. Mix well to combine. Spread bean mixture evenly over partially baked crust. Sprinkle mozzarella cheese over top. Continue baking 10 to 15 minutes or until crust is golden brown and cheese is melted. Place pizza pan on a wire rack and let set for 5 minutes. Cut into 8 wedges.

Each serving equals:

HE: 1¾ Protein • 1 Bread • ½ Vegetable •
2 Optional Calories

---

220 Calories • 8 gm Fat • 12 gm Protein •
25 gm Carbohydrate • 494 mg Sodium •
166 mg Calcium • 3 gm Fiber

DIABETIC: 1½ Starch • 1 Meat • ½ Vegetable

Mediterranean Spaghetti Skillet ❄

If the only way you usually enjoy feta cheese is as part of a Greek salad, try stirring it into this skillet spaghetti dish that's tangy with the tastes of all the countries bordering this great sea! You'll feel as if you've cruised from Spain and Italy all the way to the islands.

❍   Serves 4 (1 cup)

> 2 tablespoons Kraft Fat Free Italian Dressing
> 1½ cups diced unpeeled zucchini
> ½ cup chopped onion
> 1¾ cups (one 15-ounce can) Hunt's Tomato Sauce
> ¼ cup (1-ounce) sliced ripe olives
> ½ cup (one 2.5-ounce jar) sliced mushrooms, drained
> 2 cups hot cooked spaghetti, rinsed and drained
> ⅓ cup (1½ ounces) crumbled feta cheese

In a large skillet, combine Italian dressing, zucchini, and onion. Cook over medium heat until vegetables are tender, stirring often. Stir in tomato sauce, olives, mushrooms, and spaghetti. Add feta cheese. Mix well to combine. Lower heat and simmer for 5 minutes, or until mixture is heated through, stirring often.

HINT: 1½ cups broken uncooked spaghetti usually cooks to about 2 cups.

Each serving equals:

HE: 3 Vegetable • 1 Bread • ½ Protein • ¼ Fat • 2 Optional Calories

---

175 Calories • 3 gm Fat • 7 gm Protein • 30 gm Carbohydrate • 936 mg Sodium • 177 mg Calcium • 3 gm Fiber

---

DIABETIC: 3 Vegetable • 1 Starch • ½ Meat

Cabbage–Kidney Bean Bake

Meatless main dishes can be as varied as you like, drawing their protein from beans, vegetables, eggs, and cheeses. This inventive baked cabbage and bean dish is also wonderfully high in fiber *and* flavor!   ☻   Serves 4

2½ cups shredded cabbage
½ cup chunky salsa (mild, medium, or hot)
1 teaspoon dried parsley flakes
1 (10¾-ounce) can Healthy Request Tomato Soup
10 ounces (one 16-ounce can) red kidney beans, rinsed and
  drained
2 cups hot cooked noodles, rinsed and drained
⅓ cup (1½ ounces) shredded Kraft reduced-fat Cheddar cheese

Preheat oven to 350 degrees. Spray an 8-by-8-inch baking dish with butter-flavored cooking spray. In a large skillet sprayed with butter-flavored cooking spray, sauté cabbage for 5 minutes or just until tender. Stir in salsa, parsley flakes, and tomato soup. Add kidney beans and noodles. Mix well to combine. Pour mixture into prepared baking dish. Sprinkle Cheddar cheese evenly over top. Bake for 20 minutes. Place baking dish on a wire rack and let set for 5 minutes. Divide into 4 servings.

HINT: 1¾ cups uncooked noodles usually cooks to about 2 cups.

Each serving equals:

HE: 1¾ Protein • 1½ Vegetable • 1 Bread •
½ Slider • 5 Optional Calories

---

260 Calories • 4 gm Fat • 12 gm Protein •
44 gm Carbohydrate • 444 mg Sodium •
167 mg Calcium • 7 gm Fiber

DIABETIC: 2½ Starch • 1 Meat • 1 Vegetable

Mexican Corn Bake

Imagine stirring up this rich baked corn dish in a couple of minutes, then enjoying almost an hour of relaxation before dinner is served! If "south of the border" is your geographical home, then this recipe should be a regular in your repertoire.   ◐   Serves 8

¾ cup Bisquick Reduced Fat Baking Mix
⅔ cup Carnation Nonfat Dry Milk Powder
1 egg or equivalent in egg substitute
1 cup (one 8-ounce can) cream-style corn
½ cup chunky salsa (mild, medium, or hot)
1 cup frozen whole-kernel corn
½ cup canned chopped green chilies, drained (optional)
⅔ cup (2¼ ounces) shredded Kraft reduced-fat Cheddar cheese

Preheat oven to 350 degrees. Spray an 8-by-8-inch baking dish with olive oil-flavored cooking spray. In a large bowl, combine dry baking mix and dry milk powder. Add egg, cream-style corn, and salsa. Mix well to combine. Stir in frozen corn and green chilies. Pour mixture into prepared baking dish. Evenly sprinkle Cheddar cheese over top. Bake for 40 to 45 minutes. Place baking dish on a wire rack and let set for 5 minutes. Divide into 8 servings.

Each serving equals:

HE: 1 Bread • ½ Protein • ¼ Vegetable •
¼ Skim Milk

134 Calories • 2 gm Fat • 7 gm Protein •
22 gm Carbohydrate • 438 mg Sodium •
175 mg Calcium • 2 gm Fiber

DIABETIC: 1½ Starch • ½ Meat

Grande Macaroni and Cheese

Here's a dish sure to elicit cries of "Olé! Hooray!" as you place this cozy casserole with a Mexican flair on your dinner table! I've spiced up traditional mac and cheese in this recipe that Cliff voted was one of his newest favorites.   ☻   Serves 6

> 1 (10¾-ounce) can Healthy Request Cream of Mushroom Soup
> ¾ cup chunky salsa (mild, medium, or hot)
> 1 teaspoon dried parsley flakes
> 1 teaspoon chili seasoning
> 1½ cups (6 ounces) shredded Kraft reduced-fat Cheddar cheese
> 3 cups hot cooked elbow macaroni, rinsed and drained

Preheat oven to 350 degrees. Spray an 8-by-8-inch baking dish with olive oil–flavored cooking spray. In a large skillet, combine mushroom soup, salsa, parsley flakes, and chili seasoning. Stir in Cheddar cheese. Cook over medium heat until cheese melts, stirring often. Add macaroni. Mix well to combine. Pour mixture into prepared baking dish. Bake for 30 to 35 minutes. Place baking dish on a wire rack and let set for 5 minutes. Divide into 6 servings.

HINT: 2¼ cups uncooked macaroni usually cooks to about 3 cups.

Each serving equals:

HE: 1⅓ Protein • 1 Bread • ¼ Vegetable •
¼ Slider • 10 Optional Calories

202 Calories • 6 gm Fat • 11 gm Protein •
26 gm Carbohydrate • 549 mg Sodium •
266 mg Calcium • 1 gm Fiber

DIABETIC: 1½ Starch • 1 Meat

Easy Tuna Noodle Casserole

Doesn't every family have at least one tuna casserole to call its own? I like this easy but oh-so-tasty version that skips the traditional potato chip topping for luscious cheese slices instead.

❍ Serves 4

2 cups hot cooked noodles, rinsed and drained
1 (6-ounce) can white tuna, packed in water, drained and flaked
½ cup (one 2.5-ounce jar) sliced mushrooms, drained
2 cups (one 16-ounce can) cut green beans, rinsed and drained
1 (10¾-ounce) can Healthy Request Cream of Mushroom Soup
1 teaspoon dried onion flakes
1 teaspoon dried parsley flakes
⅛ teaspoon black pepper
4 (¾-ounce) slices Kraft reduced-fat American cheese

Preheat oven to 350 degrees. Spray an 8-by-8-inch baking dish with butter-flavored cooking spray. In a large bowl, combine noodles, tuna, mushrooms, and green beans. Add mushroom soup, onion flakes, parsley flakes, and black pepper. Mix well to combine. Spread mixture into prepared baking dish. Evenly arrange American cheese slices over top. Bake for 25 to 30 minutes. Place baking dish on a wire rack and let set for 5 minutes. Divide into 4 servings.

HINT: 1¾ cups uncooked noodles usually cooks to about 2 cups.

Each serving equals:

HE: 1¾ Protein • 1¼ Vegetable • 1 Bread • ½ Slider • 1 Optional Calorie

253 Calories • 5 gm Fat • 21 gm Protein • 31 gm Carbohydrate • 868 mg Sodium • 208 mg Calcium • 2 gm Fiber

DIABETIC: 2 Meat • 1½ Starch • 1 Vegetable

Veggie Baked Fish

Baking fish and a melange of vegetables together just seems to make both better! If you've never used lemon pepper, give it a try. You'll see how often it appears in my recipes—and after trying it, you'll use it all the time too. ● Serves 2

1 cup unpeeled sliced zucchini
1/2 cup sliced green bell pepper
1 cup peeled and sliced fresh tomatoes
1/2 cup sliced onion
8 ounces white fish, cut into 2 pieces
1/2 teaspoon lemon pepper
1/4 cup water
2 teaspoons reduced-calorie margarine
1/8 teaspoon paprika

Preheat oven to 350 degrees. Place half of zucchini, green pepper, tomatoes, and onion in an 8-by-8-inch baking dish. Place fish pieces over vegetables. Sprinkle lemon pepper over top. Cover fish with remaining vegetables. Pour water over vegetables. Spoon 1 teaspoon margarine over top of each piece of fish and evenly sprinkle paprika over top. Bake for 20 to 25 minutes. Place baking dish on a wire rack and let set for 5 minutes.

Each serving equals:

HE: 3 Vegetable • 2 Protein • 1/2 Fat

134 Calories • 2 gm Fat • 18 gm Protein •
11 gm Carbohydrate • 122 mg Sodium •
68 mg Calcium • 3 gm Fiber

DIABETIC: 3 Meat • 2 Vegetable • 1/2 Fat

Fish Fillets au Gratin

This dish always looks fancy—it must be the topping of cheese and bread crumbs that does it! This is a terrific healthy choice when you're grilling outdoors and want something other than burgers or chicken.   ☻   Serves 4

> *16 ounces white fish, cut into 4 pieces*
> *6 tablespoons (1½ ounces) dried fine bread crumbs*
> *¾ cup (3 ounces) shredded Kraft reduced-fat Cheddar cheese*
> *¼ teaspoon lemon pepper*
> *1 teaspoon dried parsley flakes*

Cut four (12-inch) squares of aluminum foil. Lightly spray each with butter-flavored cooking spray. Place fish pieces on foil. In a small bowl, combine bread crumbs, Cheddar cheese, lemon pepper, and parsley flakes. Evenly sprinkle bread mixture over fish pieces. Seal packets. Place packets on a grill and cook for 20 to 25 minutes or place packets on a baking sheet and bake for 30 minutes in a preheated 350-degree oven.

Each serving equals:

HE: 3 Protein • ½ Bread

189 Calories • 5 gm fat • 28 gm Protein • 8 gm Carbohydrate • 352 mg Sodium • 206 mg Calcium • 0 gm Fiber

DIABETIC: 4 Meat • ½ Starch

Cajun Fish Skillet

Because of all the health benefits we've heard about, most people have been trying to eat more fish, but many people aren't sure how to cook it so it turns out truly flavorful. This quick and slightly spicy Cajun version is simple but sensationally good.

○ Serves 4

> ½ cup chopped green bell pepper
> ½ cup chopped onion
> 1 (10¾-ounce) can Healthy Request Tomato Soup
> ¼ cup water
> 1 teaspoon Cajun seasoning
> 1 teaspoon dried parsley flakes
> 16 ounces white fish, cut into 4 pieces

In a large skillet sprayed with butter-flavored cooking spray, sauté green pepper and onion for 5 minutes or until tender. Stir in tomato soup, water, Cajun seasoning, and parsley flakes. Bring mixture to a boil. Evenly arrange fish pieces in skillet. Lower heat, cover, and simmer for 10 minutes or until fish flakes easily. When serving, evenly spoon sauce over fish pieces.

Each serving equals:

HE: 1½ Protein • ½ Vegetable • ½ Slider • 5 Optional Calories

---

158 Calories • 2 gm Fat • 23 gm Protein •
12 gm Carbohydrate • 323 mg Sodium •
58 mg Calcium • 1 gm Fiber

DIABETIC: 3 Meat • 1 Starch

Cinque Terre Shrimp Pasta

While having dinner in New York with my editor, John Duff, I spotted this tasty dish on the menu. It was so flavorful that I immediately stirred it up in my mind, then re-created it when I returned home. I'm happy to report it tasted every bit as good in DeWitt as it did in New York. In case you're wondering about this recipe's unusual name, it's the name of the restaurant.

☾ Serves 4 (1¼ cups)

> ¼ cup finely chopped onion
>
> 1¾ cups (one 14½-ounce can) stewed tomatoes, coarsely chopped and undrained
>
> ¼ cup Heinz Light Harvest Ketchup or any reduced-sodium ketchup
>
> 1 teaspoon Italian seasoning
>
> ¼ cup (¾ ounce) grated Kraft fat-free Parmesan cheese
>
> 1½ cups hot cooked noodles, rinsed and drained
>
> 1 cup frozen whole-kernel corn, thawed
>
> 1 (4.5-ounce drained weight) can small shrimp, rinsed and drained
>
> 1 tablespoon chopped fresh parsley or 1 teaspoon dried parsley flakes

In a large skillet sprayed with butter-flavored cooking spray, sauté onion for 5 minutes or until tender. Stir in undrained stewed tomatoes, ketchup, Italian seasoning, and Parmesan cheese. Add noodles, corn, shrimp, and parsley. Mix well to combine. Lower heat and simmer for 10 minutes, stirring occasionally.

HINTS: 1. 1¼ cups uncooked noodles usually cooks to about 1½ cups.
2. Thaw corn by placing in a colander and rinsing under hot water for one minute.

Each serving equals:

HE: 1⅓ Protein • 1¼ Bread • 1 Vegetable •
10 Optional Calories

205 Calories • 1 gm Fat • 13 gm Protein •
36 gm Carbohydrate • 571 mg Sodium •
86 mg Calcium • 3 gm Fiber

DIABETIC: 2 Starch • 1½ Meat • 1 Vegetable

White Fish with Shrimp Sauce

It sounds almost decadent, doesn't it, topping your fish fillets with a sauce that stars shrimp! This is a perfect example of how today's healthy soups (along with a little advice from me!) can help turn you into a star chef. Whether you do your fishing at the local grocery or favorite fishing hole, this "catch of the day" will win you over. ☻ Serves 4

> 16 ounces white fish, cut into 4 pieces
> 1 (10¾-ounce) can Healthy Request Cream of Mushroom Soup
> 1 (4.5-ounce drained weight) can small shrimp, rinsed and drained
> 1 teaspoon seafood seasoning

Preheat oven to 400 degrees. Spray an 8-by-8-inch baking dish with butter-flavored cooking spray. Arrange fish pieces in prepared baking dish. Lightly spray tops of fish pieces with butter-flavored cooking spray. Bake for 20 minutes. Reduce heat to 350 degrees. In a medium bowl, combine mushroom soup, shrimp, and seafood seasoning. Evenly spoon soup mixture over partially baked fish. Continue baking for 15 minutes. When serving, evenly spoon sauce over fish pieces.

Each serving equals:

HE: 2½ Protein • ½ Slider • 1 Optional Calorie

171 Calories • 3 gm Fat • 29 gm Protein •
7 gm Carbohydrate • 446 mg Sodium •
112 mg Calcium • 0 gm Fiber

DIABETIC: 4 Meat • ½ Starch

Chicken and Dumplings

What more classic "comfort food" dish could there be than this one, which graced more Sunday dinner tables than almost any other Midwest meal? And just think, you can put the ingredients in your slow cooker before you head off to church, then add the dumplings when you return—and in less than an hour, you've got a scrumptious dish that tastes like home! ☻ Serves 4

1½ cups (8 ounces) diced cooked chicken breast
1⅓ cups skim milk☆
1 (10¾-ounce) can Healthy Request Cream of Chicken Soup
1 cup (one 8-ounce can) cut green beans, rinsed and drained
1 cup (one 8-ounce can) cut carrots, rinsed and drained
½ teaspoon poultry seasoning
¾ cup Bisquick Reduced Fat Baking Mix
1 teaspoon dried parsley flakes

In a slow cooker container, combine chicken, 1 cup skim milk, chicken soup, green beans, carrots, and poultry seasoning. Cover and cook on LOW for 3 to 4 hours. In a medium bowl, combine baking mix, remaining ⅓ cup skim milk, and parsley flakes. Mix well. Drop by spoonful into cooked mixture to form 4 dumplings. Cover and continue cooking on LOW for 45 to 50 minutes. For each serving, place 1 dumpling on a serving plate and spoon about ¾ cup chicken mixture over top.

Each serving equals:

HE: 2 Protein • 1 Vegetable • 1 Bread •
¼ Skim Milk • ½ Slider • 13 Optional Calories

265 Calories • 5 gm Fat • 24 gm Protein •
31 gm Carbohydrate • 661 mg Sodium •
146 mg Calcium • 1 gm Fiber

DIABETIC: 2 Meat • 2 Starch • 1 Vegetable

Company Chicken and Rice Casserole

Were you stuck in the kitchen fixing dinner the last time you invited guests over? We've all had that happen, but here's a recipe that will let you enjoy your company and still present a wonderful meal. This also freezes well, so if you've got leftovers, you can defrost them later and treat yourself like company!

○ Serves 4

> 1½ cups (8 ounces) diced cooked chicken breast
> 1 cup cold cooked rice
> ¾ cup chopped celery
> ¼ cup chopped onion
> ½ cup (one 2.5-ounce jar) sliced mushrooms, drained
> ¼ cup Kraft fat-free mayonnaise
> 1 (10¾-ounce) can Healthy Request Cream of Chicken Soup
> 1 teaspoon dried parsley flakes
> 1 hard-boiled egg, chopped
> 10 Ritz Reduced Fat Crackers, made into crumbs

Preheat oven to 350 degrees. Spray an 8-by-8-inch baking dish with butter-flavored cooking spray. In a large bowl, combine chicken, rice, celery, onion, and mushrooms. Add mayonnaise, chicken soup, and parsley flakes. Mix gently to combine. Fold in egg. Spread mixture into prepared baking dish. Evenly sprinkle cracker crumbs over top. Bake for 45 minutes or until mixture is bubbly. Place baking dish on a wire rack and let set for 5 minutes. Divide into 4 servings.

HINTS: 1. ⅔ cup uncooked rice usually cooks to about 1 cup.
          2. If you want the look and feel of egg without the cholesterol, toss out the yolk and dice the white.

Each serving equals:

HE: 2¼ Protein (¼ limited) • 1 Bread • ¾ Vegetable •
½ Slider • 15 Optional Calories

254 Calories • 6 gm Fat • 23 gm Protein •
27 gm Carbohydrate • 659 mg Sodium •
41 mg Calcium • 1 gm Fiber

DIABETIC: 2 Meat • 2 Starch • ½ Vegetable

Chicken Casserole

This chicken and noodles dish tastes like the old-fashioned meals your grandma used to make, but its speedy preparation makes sense for busy people who can't spend hours in the kitchen. You'll be amazed how just a bit of flour added to evaporated skim milk transforms it into a rich, hearty sauce.   ☻   Serves 6

> 1½ cups (8 ounces) diced cooked chicken breast
> ½ cup frozen peas, thawed
> ¾ cup (3 ounces) shredded Kraft reduced-fat Cheddar cheese
> 2 cups hot cooked noodles, rinsed and drained
> ½ cup chopped onion
> ½ cup (one 2.5-ounce jar) sliced mushrooms, drained
> 2 cups (one 16-ounce can) sliced carrots, rinsed and drained
> 1½ cups (one 12-fluid-ounce can) Carnation Evaporated Skim
>   Milk
> 3 tablespoons all-purpose flour
> 1 teaspoon prepared mustard

Preheat oven to 350 degrees. Spray an 8-by-8-inch baking dish with butter-flavored cooking spray. In a large bowl, combine chicken, peas, Cheddar cheese, noodles, onion, mushrooms, and carrots. Mix well to combine. Pour chicken mixture into prepared baking dish. In a covered jar, combine evaporated skim milk and flour. Shake well to blend. Add mustard. Mix well to combine. Pour milk mixture evenly over chicken mixture. Bake for 30 to 35 minutes. Place baking dish on a wire rack and let set for 5 minutes. Divide into 6 servings.

HINTS: 1. Thaw peas by placing in a colander and rinsing under hot water for one minute.
2. 1¾ cups uncooked noodles usually cooks to about 2 cups.

Each serving equals:

HE: 2 Protein • 1 Bread • 1 Vegetable • ½ Skim Milk

240 Calories • 4 gm Fat • 24 gm Protein •
27 gm Carbohydrate • 282 mg Sodium •
311 mg Calcium • 2 gm Fiber

DIABETIC: 2 Meat • 1 Starch • 1 Vegetable •
½ Skim Milk

Chicken and Biscuit Patchwork Dinner

Did you ever think that you'd be enjoying biscuits and gravy again once you'd decided to follow a healthy lifestyle? Not all the new fat-free and reduced-fat products are truly tasty, but I'm happy to recommend the ones I've tried that are. This is comfort food at its best—and will warm you up like a cuddle in your favorite quilt!   ☻   Serves 6

1 (12-ounce) jar Heinz Fat Free Chicken Gravy

½ teaspoon poultry seasoning

1 full cup (6 ounces) diced cooked chicken breast

1¼ cups frozen cut green beans, thawed

1¼ cups frozen carrots, thawed

¼ cup frozen peas, thawed

½ cup (one 2.5-ounce jar) sliced mushrooms, drained

1 (7.5-ounce) can Pillsbury refrigerated buttermilk biscuits

Preheat oven to 400 degrees. Spray an 8-by-8-inch baking dish with butter-flavored cooking spray. In a large bowl, combine chicken gravy and poultry seasoning. Add chicken, green beans, carrots, peas, and mushrooms. Mix well to combine. Separate biscuits and cut each into 4 pieces. Add biscuit pieces to chicken mixture. Mix gently to combine. Pour mixture into prepared baking dish. Bake for 25 to 30 minutes. Place baking dish on a wire rack and let set for 5 minutes. Divide into 6 servings.

HINT: Thaw vegetables by placing in a colander and rinsing under hot water for one minute.

Each serving equals:

HE: 1 Bread • 1 Vegetable • 1 Protein • ¼ Slider •
5 Optional Calories

---

170 Calories • 2 gm Fat • 13 gm Protein •
25 gm Carbohydrate • 721 mg Sodium •
34 mg Calcium • 4 gm Fiber

DIABETIC: 1 Starch • 1 Vegetable • 1 Meat

Mexican Chicken Scallop

Here's a mouth-watering way to make just a bit of chicken feed a family of four! They won't miss the meat when they "dive" into this combination of spicy scalloped potatoes and corn that supplies plenty of chicken flavor in a dish that won't strain your budget.

☻ Serves 4

> *3 cups (10 ounces) shredded loose-packed frozen potatoes*
> *1 cup (one 8-ounce can) whole-kernel corn, rinsed and drained*
> *1 cup (5 ounces) diced cooked chicken breast*
> *½ cup chunky salsa (mild, medium, or hot)*
> *1 (10¾-ounce) can Healthy Request Cream of Chicken Soup*
> *1 teaspoon dried parsley flakes*
> *⅓ cup (1½ ounces) shredded Kraft reduced-fat Cheddar cheese*

Preheat oven to 350 degrees. Spray an 8-by-8-inch baking dish with olive oil–flavored cooking spray. In a large bowl, combine potatoes, corn, and chicken. Add salsa, chicken soup, and parsley flakes. Mix well to combine. Spread mixture into prepared baking dish. Bake for 30 minutes. Evenly sprinkle Cheddar cheese over top and continue baking for 10 minutes. Place baking dish on a wire rack and let set for 5 minutes. Divide into 4 servings.

HINT: Mr. Dell's frozen shredded potatoes are a good choice for this recipe.

Each serving equals:

HE: 1¾ Protein • 1 Bread • ¼ Vegetable • ½ Slider •
5 Optional Calories

---

220 Calories • 4 gm Fat • 17 gm Protein •
29 gm Carbohydrate • 528 mg Sodium •
118 mg Calcium • 2 gm Fiber

DIABETIC: 2 Starch • 1½ Meat

Chicken Potato Casserole

This inviting casserole is almost a shepherd's pie made with chicken, but instead of spreading the mashed potatoes on top, I've mixed it all together and added just enough Cheddar cheese to make your taste buds happy. It's a real "stick-to-your-ribs" dish, the kind Cliff loves to "taste-test" for me! ☻   Serves 4

2 cups (one 16-ounce can) Healthy Request Chicken Broth

1⅓ cups (3 ounces) instant potato flakes

⅓ cup Carnation Nonfat Dry Milk Powder

¼ teaspoon black pepper

1 full cup (6 ounces) diced cooked chicken breast

1 cup (one 8-ounce can) small peas, rinsed and drained

1 cup (one 8-ounce can) diced carrots, rinsed and drained

1 teaspoon dried parsley flakes

⅓ cup (1½ ounces) shredded Kraft reduced-fat Cheddar cheese

Preheat oven to 350 degrees. Spray an 8-by-8-inch baking dish with butter-flavored cooking spray. In a medium saucepan, bring chicken broth to a boil. Remove from heat and stir in potato flakes. Add dry milk powder and black pepper. Mix well to combine. Stir in chicken, peas, carrots, and parsley flakes. Spread mixture into prepared baking dish. Sprinkle Cheddar cheese evenly over top. Bake for 15 to 20 minutes. Place baking dish on a wire rack and let set for 5 minutes. Divide into 4 servings.

Each serving equals:

HE: 2 Protein • 1½ Bread • ½ Vegetable • ¼ Skim Milk • 15 Optional Calories

---

220 Calories • 4 gm Fat • 23 gm Protein • 23 gm Carbohydrate • 424 mg Sodium • 169 mg Calcium • 4 gm Fiber

---

DIABETIC: 2 Meat • 1½ Starch • ½ Vegetable

Chicken Pita Olé

One of the most popular ways to serve sandwich fillings these days is to wrap them in tortillas or other kinds of bread. I really like this spicy chicken blend stuffed into a pita. It's got lots and lots of flavor, provides creaminess and crunch, and will please any member of the family from age 5 to 95! ☻ Serves 4

1 full cup (6 ounces) diced cooked chicken breast
½ cup finely diced celery
½ cup chunky salsa (mild, medium, or hot)
⅓ cup Kraft fat-free mayonnaise
1 teaspoon dried parsley flakes
2 pita rounds, halved
½ cup finely shredded lettuce
2 tablespoons Kraft Fat Free Italian Dressing

In a medium bowl, combine chicken and celery. Add salsa, mayonnaise, and parsley flakes. Mix well to combine. Spoon about ½ cup chicken mixture into each pita half. In a small bowl, combine lettuce and Italian dressing. Gently mix to coat lettuce. Sprinkle about 2 tablespoons lettuce mixture over top of each pita sandwich. Serve at once or cover and refrigerate until ready to serve.

HINT: To make opening pita rounds easier, place pita halves on a paper towel and microwave on HIGH for 10 seconds. Remove and gently press open.

Each serving equals:

HE: 1½ Protein • 1 Bread • ¾ Vegetable •
15 Optional Calories

---

174 Calories • 2 gm Fat • 16 gm Protein •
23 gm Carbohydrate • 566 mg Sodium •
81 mg Calcium • 1 gm Fiber

DIABETIC: 1½ Meat • 1 Starch • 1 Vegetable

Quick Chicken and Rice

A luscious chicken and rice dinner in about fifteen minutes—can it be done? Yes! This skillet supper tastes so cozy and warm, you'll wonder why every dinner can't be prepared this fast!

● Serves 4 (1 cup)

½ cup finely chopped onion
1½ cups (8 ounces) diced cooked chicken breast
1 (12-ounce) jar Heinz Fat Free Chicken Gravy
1 cup (one 8-ounce can) peas, undrained
⅔ cup (2 ounces) uncooked Minute Rice
1 teaspoon dried parsley flakes

In a large skillet sprayed with butter-flavored cooking spray, sauté onion for 5 minutes or until tender. Stir in chicken, chicken gravy, and undrained peas. Bring mixture to a boil. Add uncooked rice and parsley flakes. Mix well to combine. Remove from heat, cover, and let set for 5 minutes. Mix well again just before serving.

Each serving equals:

HE: 2 Protein • 1 Bread • ¼ Vegetable •
15 Optional Calories

174 Calories • 2 gm Fat • 22 gm Protein •
17 gm Carbohydrate • 535 mg Sodium •
42 mg Calcium • 3 gm Fiber

DIABETIC: 2 Meat • 1 Starch

Fiesta Turkey and Noodles

Here's a great way to use up leftover holiday turkey that's savory and satisfying to the eye as well as the tummy! Unless everyone enjoys mouth-tingling spiciness, I recommend using a mild salsa, then offering hotter blends to be added at the table by anyone who wants more "heat!"   ☺   Serves 4 (1 cup)

> 1½ cups (8 ounces) diced cooked turkey breast
> 1 (12-ounce) jar Heinz Fat Free Turkey or Chicken Gravy
> ½ cup chunky salsa (mild, medium, or hot)
> ½ cup (one 2.5-ounce jar) sliced mushrooms, drained
> 1 teaspoon dried parsley flakes
> 2 cups hot cooked noodles, rinsed and drained

In a large skillet sprayed with butter-flavored cooking spray, combine turkey and gravy. Stir in salsa, mushrooms, and parsley flakes. Bring mixture to a boil. Add noodles. Mix well to combine. Lower heat and simmer for 5 minutes, or until mixture is heated through, stirring occasionally.

HINT: 1¾ cups uncooked noodles usually cooks to about 2 cups.

Each serving equals:

HE: 2 Protein • 1 Bread • ½ Vegetable • ¼ Slider • 3 Optional Calories

---

223 Calories • 3 gm Fat • 23 gm Protein • 26 gm Carbohydrate • 732 mg Sodium • 79 mg Calcium • 2 gm Fiber

---

DIABETIC: 2 Meat • 1½ Starch • 1 Vegetable

Turkey Rice Skillet

It almost seems impossible to feed six people on half a pound of turkey, but this yummy stovetop sensation will make a believer out of everyone! It's a terrific choice for a Sunday supper, or for any weeknight when there's just no time to cook.

● Serves 6 (1 cup)

½ cup chopped onion
1 cup finely chopped celery
1½ cups (8 ounces) diced cooked turkey breast
½ cup (one 2.5-ounce jar) sliced mushrooms, drained
1 (10¾-ounce) can Healthy Request Cream of Chicken Soup
1 cup skim milk
1 teaspoon poultry seasoning
1 teaspoon dried parsley flakes
½ teaspoon black pepper
1⅓ cups (4 ounces) uncooked Minute Rice

In a large skillet sprayed with butter-flavored cooking spray, sauté onion and celery for 5 minutes or until tender. Stir in turkey and mushrooms. Add chicken soup, skim milk, poultry seasoning, parsley flakes, and black pepper. Mix well to combine. Bring mixture to a boil. Stir in uncooked rice. Remove from heat, cover, and let set for 5 minutes. Mix well again just before serving.

Each serving equals:

HE: 2 Protein • 1 Bread • 1 Vegetable •
¼ Skim Milk • ½ Slider • 5 Optional Calories

190 Calories • 2 gm Fat • 16 gm Protein •
27 gm Carbohydrate • 324 mg Sodium •
74 mg Calcium • 1 gm Fiber

DIABETIC: 2 Meat • 1½ Starch • ½ Vegetable

Plymouth Rock Pizza

Tired of serving holiday leftovers? Feel like the next sound out of your mouth might be a gobble? Don't despair—here's a totally original way to serve turkey that will make you smack your lips in delight. ☻ Serves 8

> 1 (4-serving) package JELL-O sugar-free vanilla cook-and-serve pudding mix
> 1 cup Ocean Spray reduced-calorie cranberry juice cocktail
> 3 cups fresh or frozen cranberries
> 1 (8-ounce) package Philadelphia fat-free cream cheese
> 1 (11-ounce) can Pillsbury refrigerated French bread
> 1½ cups (8 ounces) diced cooked turkey breast
> ½ cup (2 ounces) chopped walnuts

Preheat oven to 415 degrees. In a large saucepan, combine dry pudding mix and cranberry juice cocktail. Stir in cranberries. Cook over medium heat until mixture starts to boil and cranberries soften, stirring constantly. Remove from heat. Stir in cream cheese. Place saucepan on a wire rack and allow to cool while preparing crust. Meanwhile, unroll French loaf and pat into a 10-by-15-inch rimmed baking pan. Bake for 10 minutes. Evenly spread cranberry mixture over partially baked crust. Sprinkle turkey and walnuts evenly over top. Continue baking for 8 to 10 minutes or until crust is golden brown. Place baking pan on a wire rack and let set for 5 minutes. Cut into 8 servings.

Each serving equals:

HE: 1¾ Protein • 1 Bread • ½ Fat • ½ Fruit • 10 Optional Calories

---

243 Calories • 7 gm Fat • 17 gm Protein • 28 gm Carbohydrate • 499 mg Sodium • 14 mg Calcium • 2 gm Fiber

---

DIABETIC: 2 Starch/Carbohydrate • 1½ Meat • ½ Fat

Fancy Fiesta Skillet

Did you know that salsa is the most popular condiment in America these days? It's true! And why not, when just a half cup or so can make every dish a celebration of flavor and fun? This appetizing combo is easy enough for your teens to prepare—or even a husband! But it tastes like a special treat!

○ Serves 4 (1 cup)

> 8 ounces ground 90% lean turkey or beef
> ½ cup chunky salsa (mild, medium, or hot)
> 1 (12-ounce) jar Heinz Fat Free Beef Gravy
> 2 cups hot cooked noodles, rinsed and drained
> 1 teaspoon dried parsley flakes

In a large skillet sprayed with olive oil–flavored cooking spray, brown meat. Stir in salsa and beef gravy. Add noodles and parsley flakes. Mix well to combine. Lower heat and simmer for 10 minutes, stirring occasionally.

HINT: 1¾ cups uncooked noodles usually cooks to about 2 cups.

Each serving equals:

HE: 1½ Protein • 1 Bread • ¼ Vegetable •
¼ Slider • 3 Optional Calories

---

214 Calories • 6 gm Fat • 15 gm Protein •
25 gm Carbohydrate • 666 mg Sodium •
51 mg Calcium • 1 gm Fiber

DIABETIC: 1½ Meat • 1½ Starch • ½ Vegetable

Macaroni Skillet Dinner

Maybe you're snowed in, and the only thing in your fridge is a pound of ground beef. Maybe you just can't bear the idea of getting in the car again to go to the store. Here's a perfect "pantry" meal that you can stir up in minutes with a minimum of effort—and it delivers plenty of sizzle!   ❂   Serves 6 (1 cup)

> 16 ounces ground 90% lean turkey or beef
> 1 cup (one 8-ounce can) Hunt's Tomato Sauce
> ½ cup water
> 1 tablespoon Worcestershire sauce
> 1 tablespoon dried onion flakes
> 1 teaspoon dried parsley flakes
> ¼ teaspoon black pepper
> ¾ cup (3 ounces) shredded Kraft reduced-fat Cheddar
>   cheese
> 2 cups hot cooked elbow macaroni, rinsed and drained
> 1 cup frozen whole-kernel corn, thawed
> 2 cups (one 16-ounce can) French-style green beans, rinsed and
>   drained

In a large skillet sprayed with butter-flavored cooking spray, brown meat. Stir in tomato sauce, water, Worcestershire sauce, onion flakes, parsley flakes, and black pepper. Add Cheddar cheese. Mix well to combine. Stir in macaroni, corn, and green beans. Lower heat, cover, and simmer for 10 minutes, stirring occasionally.

HINTS: 1. 1¾ cups uncooked macaroni usually cooks to about 2 cups.
    2. Thaw corn by placing in a colander and rinsing under hot water for one minute.

Each serving equals:

HE: 2⅔ Protein • 1⅓ Vegetable • 1 Bread

256 Calories • 8 gm Fat • 21 gm Protein •
25 gm Carbohydrate • 488 mg Sodium •
115 mg Calcium • 3 gm Fiber

DIABETIC: 2½ Meat • 1 Vegetable • 1 Starch

Comfort Biscuits and Gravy

One of the most popular dishes in my first cookbook was Truck-stop Biscuits and Gravy. Since then, everyone keeps asking me for more ways to get the irresistible flavor of sausage and gravy without the calories and fat. Let me "comfort" you with this tasty dish that will fool your taste buds—and make you pat your tummy with pleasure.   ☻   Serves 6

> 16 ounces ground 90% lean turkey or beef
> ½ teaspoon poultry seasoning
> ¼ teaspoon ground sage
> ¼ teaspoon garlic powder
> 1 (10¾-ounce) can Healthy Request Cream of Mushroom
>   Soup
> ⅔ cup Carnation Nonfat Dry Milk Powder
> 1 cup water
> 1 (8-ounce) package Philadelphia fat-free cream cheese
> 1 (7.5-ounce) can Pillsbury refrigerated buttermilk biscuits

Preheat oven to 415 degrees. Spray an 8-by-8-inch baking dish with butter-flavored cooking spray. In a large skillet sprayed with butter-flavored cooking spray, brown meat. Stir in poultry seasoning, sage, and garlic powder. In a small bowl, combine mushroom soup, dry milk powder, and water. Add soup mixture to meat mixture. Mix well to combine. Stir in cream cheese. Continue cooking until cream cheese melts and mixture is heated through, stirring constantly. Pour meat mixture into prepared baking dish. Separate biscuits and cut each into 4 pieces. Evenly sprinkle biscuit pieces over top of meat mixture. Lightly spray top with butter-flavored cooking spray. Bake for 15 to 20 minutes or until golden brown. Place baking dish on a wire rack and let set for 5 minutes. Divide into 6 servings.

Each serving equals:

HE: 2⅔ Protein • 1¼ Bread • ¼ Skim Milk • ¼ Slider • 8 Optional Calories

272 Calories • 8 gm Fat • 24 gm Protein • 26 gm Carbohydrate • 842 mg Sodium • 126 mg Calcium • 2 gm Fiber

DIABETIC: 2½ Meat • 2 Starch

Emerald Isle Skillet

My Irish heritage turns up in many of my recipes, and this one is no exception. Starring that Irish staple, the potato, as well as some St. Paddy's Day cabbage, this dish is a stovetop stunner that's almost as good as a free ticket on Aer Lingus and a trip to County Mayo!

● Serves 4 (1 cup)

> 8 ounces ground 90% lean turkey or beef
> ½ cup chopped onion
> 2½ cups shredded cabbage
> ½ cup (one 2.5-ounce jar) sliced mushrooms, drained
> 2½ cups (12 ounces) diced cooked potatoes
> 1 (10¾-ounce) can Healthy Request Cream of Mushroom Soup
> ¼ teaspoon black pepper

In a large skillet sprayed with butter-flavored cooking spray, brown meat, onion, and cabbage. Add mushrooms, potatoes, mushroom soup, and black pepper. Mix well to combine. Lower heat and simmer for 5 minutes, or until mixture is heated through, stirring occasionally.

Each serving equals:

HE: 1¾ Vegetable • 1½ Protein • 1 Bread •
½ Slider • 1 Optional Calorie

---

218 Calories • 6 gm Fat • 13 gm Protein •
28 gm Carbohydrate • 448 mg Sodium •
82 mg Calcium • 3 gm Fiber

DIABETIC: 1½ Starch • 1½ Meat • 1 Vegetable

Tom's Celery Hamburger Milk Gravy Stroganoff

It's hard to believe that my "baby" is now a married man, but I'll never stop creating hamburger milk gravy recipes without Tommy in mind! This creamy dish invites you to join him on the bandwagon and cheer its lusciousness. (Angie, don't let him have milk gravy *every day*, okay?)   ☻   Serves 4

8 ounces ground 90% lean turkey or beef
1 cup finely chopped celery
1 (10¾-ounce) can Healthy Request Cream of Mushroom Soup
1⅓ cups skim milk
½ cup (one 2.5-ounce jar) sliced mushrooms, drained
⅛ teaspoon black pepper
2 cups hot cooked noodles, rinsed and drained

In a large skillet sprayed with butter-flavored cooking spray, brown meat and celery. Stir in mushroom soup and skim milk. Add mushrooms and black pepper. Mix well to combine. Lower heat and simmer for 5 minutes, stirring occasionally. For each serving, place ½ cup noodles on a plate and spoon about ¾ cup gravy mixture over top.

HINT: 1¾ cups uncooked noodles usually cooks to about 2 cups.

Each serving equals:

HE: 1½ Protein • 1 Bread • ¾ Vegetable •
⅓ Skim Milk • ½ Slider • 1 Optional Calorie

255 Calories • 7 gm Fat • 17 gm Protein •
31 gm Carbohydrate • 310 mg Sodium •
174 mg Calcium • 2 gm Fiber

DIABETIC: 2 Starch • 1½ Meat • ½ Vegetable

Ranchero Shepherd's Pie

There are convenience foods, and then there are the convenience foods I just love—including instant mashed potatoes! They're a quick cook's dream come true because they're so versatile, and they just get better and better when you mix them with a little yogurt or cheese. There's something spectacular about a meat pie topped with mashed potatoes, don't you think?   ☻   Serves 6

> 8 ounces ground 90% lean turkey or beef
> ½ cup chunky salsa (mild, medium, or hot)
> 1 cup (one 8-ounce can) Hunt's Tomato Sauce
> 1 tablespoon Brown Sugar Twin
> 2 cups (one 16-ounce can) French-style green beans, rinsed and
>   drained
> ¾ cup (3 ounces) shredded Kraft reduced-fat Cheddar cheese☆
> 2 cups water
> 2 cups (4½ ounces) instant potato flakes
> ⅓ cup Carnation Nonfat Dry Milk Powder
> ¾ cup Yoplait plain fat-free yogurt
> 1 teaspoon dried parsley flakes
> 1 teaspoon chili seasoning
> ¼ teaspoon black pepper

Preheat oven to 375 degrees. Spray an 8-by-8-inch baking dish with olive oil–flavored cooking spray. In a large skillet sprayed with olive oil–flavored cooking spray, brown meat. Stir in salsa, tomato sauce, and Brown Sugar Twin. Add green beans and half of the Cheddar cheese. Mix well to combine. Pour mixture into prepared baking dish. In a medium saucepan, bring water to a boil. Remove from heat. Stir in potato flakes and dry milk powder. Add yogurt, parsley flakes, chili seasoning, black pepper, and remaining Cheddar cheese. Mix gently with a fork. Spread potato mixture evenly over meat mixture. Bake for 20 to 25 minutes. Place baking dish on a wire rack and let set for 5 minutes. Divide into 6 servings.

Each serving equals:

HE: 1⅔ Protein • 1½ Vegetable • 1 Bread •
⅓ Skim Milk • 1 Optional Calorie

193 Calories • 5 gm Fat • 15 gm Protein •
22 gm Carbohydrate • 554 mg Sodium •
239 mg Calcium • 2 gm Fiber

DIABETIC: 1½ Meat • 1½ Vegetable • 1 Starch

Meat Squares with Creamed Potato Topping

For anyone who's struggled with diets for many years, a dish topped with creamy potatoes often seems like an incredible splurge. Add some fat-free sour cream, and you may just think you've gone to culinary heaven. But it's no miracle, just smart and healthy cooking that finally gives you the tastes you love! ☻ Serves 4

> 8 ounces ground 90% lean turkey or beef
>
> ½ cup (one 2.5-ounce jar) sliced mushrooms, drained
>
> 3 tablespoons (¾ ounce) dried fine bread crumbs
>
> 2 tablespoons skim milk
>
> ¼ teaspoon black pepper
>
> 1¼ cups water
>
> 1 cup (2¼ ounces) instant potato flakes
>
> ⅓ cup Carnation Nonfat Dry Milk Powder
>
> 2 tablespoons Land O Lakes no-fat sour cream
>
> 1 teaspoon dried parsley flakes
>
> 1 teaspoon chili seasoning
>
> ⅓ cup (1½ ounces) shredded Kraft reduced-fat Cheddar cheese
>
> 1 tablespoon Hormel Bacon Bits

Preheat oven to 350 degrees. Spray an 8-by-8-inch baking dish with butter-flavored cooking spray. In a medium bowl, combine meat, mushrooms, and bread crumbs. Add skim milk and black pepper. Mix well to combine. Pat mixture into prepared baking dish. Bake for 30 minutes. Meanwhile, in a medium saucepan, bring water to a boil. Remove from heat. Stir in potato flakes, dry milk powder, and sour cream. Add parsley flakes and chili seasoning. Fluff well with a fork. Spread potato mixture evenly over partially baked meat mixture. Sprinkle Cheddar cheese and bacon bits evenly over top. Continue baking for 15 minutes. Place baking dish on a wire rack and let set for 5 minutes. Divide into 4 servings.

Each serving equals:

HE: 2 Protein • 1 Bread • ¼ Vegetable • ¼ Skim Milk

211 Calories • 7 gm Fat • 18 gm Protein •
19 gm Carbohydrate • 386 mg Sodium •
174 mg Calcium • 1 gm Fiber

DIABETIC: 2 Meat • 1 Starch • ½ Skim Milk

Ranchero Meatloaf

Meatloaf is one of my favorite kitchen "mysteries," because each and every one has a formula that somehow cooks up a little differently—and pleases the palate in a fresh way! I made this one a little bit sweet and a little bit tangy, then topped it with melted cheese. Isn't this kind of kitchen chemistry fun?   ☻   Serves 6

16 ounces ground 90% lean turkey or beef

14 small fat-free saltine crackers, made into crumbs

1 cup (one 8-ounce can) Hunt's Tomato Sauce☆

1 teaspoon chili seasoning

¼ cup chunky salsa (mild, medium, or hot)

1 tablespoon Brown Sugar Twin

⅓ cup (1½ ounces) shredded Kraft reduced-fat Cheddar cheese

Preheat oven to 350 degrees. Spray an 8-by-8-inch baking dish with butter-flavored cooking spray. In a medium bowl, combine meat, cracker crumbs, ¼ cup tomato sauce, and chili seasoning. Mix well to combine. Pat mixture into prepared baking dish. In a small bowl, combine remaining ¾ cup tomato sauce, salsa, and Brown Sugar Twin. Spread mixture evenly over top of meatloaf. Bake for 40 minutes. Sprinkle Cheddar cheese evenly over top of partially baked meatloaf. Continue baking 10 minutes longer or until cheese melts. Place baking dish on a wire rack and let set for 5 minutes. Cut into 6 servings.

Each serving equals:

HE: 2⅓ Protein • ¾ Vegetable • ⅓ Bread •
1 Optional Calorie

159 Calories • 7 gm Fat • 16 gm Protein •
8 gm Carbohydrate • 456 mg Sodium •
70 mg Calcium • 1 gm Fiber

DIABETIC: 2 Meat • 1 Vegetable

Florentine Meatloaf

Spinach is at the heart of any dish called "Florentine," and this flavorful meatloaf is an especially savory one. I think you'll find its unique blend of mozzarella and Parmesan remarkably tasty. If you can't manage a trip to Italy this year, why not dine *al fresco* on an entree inspired by the exquisite city of Florence? ◐ Serves 6

> 1 (10-ounce) package frozen cut spinach, thawed and thoroughly
>   drained
> 16 ounces ground 90% lean turkey or beef
> 6 tablespoons (1½ ounces) dried fine bread crumbs
> ⅓ cup (1½ ounces) shredded Kraft reduced-fat mozzarella cheese
> 1 teaspoon Italian seasoning
> 1 cup (one 8-ounce can) Hunt's Tomato Sauce☆
> 1 teaspoon Sugar Twin or Sprinkle Sweet
> ¼ cup (¾ ounce) grated Kraft fat-free Parmesan cheese

Preheat oven to 350 degrees. Spray an 8-by-8-inch baking dish with olive oil–flavored cooking spray. In a large bowl, combine spinach, meat, bread crumbs, mozzarella cheese, Italian seasoning, and ½ cup tomato sauce. Mix well to combine. Pat mixture into prepared baking dish. Bake for 30 to 35 minutes. In a small bowl, combine remaining ½ cup tomato sauce, Sugar Twin, and Parmesan cheese. Evenly spoon sauce mixture over partially baked meatloaf. Continue baking for 15 minutes. Place baking dish on a wire rack and let set for 5 minutes. Cut into 6 servings.

Each serving equals:

HE: 2½ Protein • 1 Vegetable • ⅓ Bread •
2 Optional Calories

---

188 Calories • 8 gm Fat • 18 gm Protein •
11 gm Carbohydrate • 526 mg Sodium •
112 mg Calcium • 3 gm Fiber

DIABETIC: 2½ Meat • 1 Vegetable • ½ Starch

Meatball Stew

Are you one of those cooks who use the microwave mostly to reheat coffee and prepare frozen dinners? (You're not alone, of course. I've heard that most Americans do.) But I've discovered some wonderful ways to take advantage of this appliance, especially for anyone committed to living healthy. This stew retains all of its nutrients, and couldn't be easier to fix! ◑   Serves 6

> 16 ounces ground 90% lean turkey or beef
> 6 tablespoons (1½ ounces) dried fine bread crumbs
> 2 tablespoons dried onion flakes
> 2 tablespoons water
> 1 (10¾-ounce) can Healthy Request Tomato Soup☆
> 1 teaspoon dried parsley flakes
> 2 cups (one 16-ounce can) sliced carrots, rinsed and drained
> ¾ cup frozen peas, thawed
> 1 cup (one 8-ounce can) small white onions, rinsed and drained
> 10 ounces (one 16-ounce can) whole white potatoes, rinsed and
>   drained

In a large bowl, combine meat, bread crumbs, onion flakes, water, and 2 tablespoons tomato soup. Mix well to combine. Shape into 12 meatballs and arrange in a 9-inch glass pie plate. Cover and microwave on ROAST (80% power) for 9 to 12 minutes, turning dish after 5 minutes. In a 9-by-13-inch glass baking dish, combine remaining tomato soup and parsley flakes. Stir in carrots, peas, and onions. Cut potatoes in half and add to soup mixture. Gently stir in meatballs. Microwave on BAKE (60% power) for 15 to 20 minutes, stirring gently after 10 minutes. For each serving, place 2 meatballs on a plate and evenly spoon about 1 cup stew mixture over top.

HINT: Thaw peas by placing in a colander and rinsing under hot
    water for one minute.

Each serving equals:

HE: 2 Protein • 1 Bread • 1 Vegetable • ¼ Slider •
12 Optional Calories

235 Calories • 7 gm Fat • 17 gm Protein •
26 gm Carbohydrate • 304 mg Sodium •
49 mg Calcium • 4 gm Fiber

DIABETIC: 2 Meat • 1 Starch • 1 Vegetable

Impossible Runzas

In the army, they say: "The difficult we do immediately; the impossible takes a little longer." Well, when this recipe asks you to pour a blenderful of liquid over the browned meat and veggies, you'll probably mutter, "Impossible . . . I can't believe this will emerge from the oven anything but a wet mess!" In this case, the "impossible" takes just about 45 minutes, so give it a try. Your taste buds will say thanks! (Never heard of runzas? I bet soon the entire country will love this old-timey Midwestern treat!) ☻ Serves 6

> 8 ounces ground 90% lean turkey or beef
> ½ cup chopped onion
> 2½ cups purchased coleslaw mix
> 1 tablespoon chili seasoning
> ¼ teaspoon black pepper
> 1 cup water
> ⅔ cup Carnation Nonfat Dry Milk Powder
> 2 eggs or equivalent in egg substitute
> ¾ cup Bisquick Reduced Fat Baking Mix
> 1 teaspoon dried parsley flakes
> ¾ cup (3 ounces) shredded Kraft reduced-fat Cheddar cheese

Preheat oven to 350 degrees. Spray an 8-by-8-inch baking dish with butter-flavored cooking spray. In a large skillet sprayed with butter-flavored cooking spray, brown meat, onion, and coleslaw mix. Stir in chili seasoning and black pepper. Pour mixture into prepared baking dish. In a blender container, combine water, dry milk powder, and eggs. Cover and process on HIGH for 10 seconds. Add baking mix, parsley flakes, and Cheddar cheese. Cover and process on HIGH an additional 10 seconds. Pour mixture evenly over meat mixture. Bake for 35 to 40 minutes. Place baking dish on a wire rack and let set for 5 minutes. Cut into 6 servings.

HINT: 2 cups shredded cabbage and ½ cup shredded carrots may be used in place of purchased coleslaw mix.

Each serving equals:

HE: 2 Protein (⅓ limited) • 1 Vegetable • ⅔ Bread •
⅔ Skim Milk

---

216 Calories • 8 gm Fat • 17 gm Protein •
19 gm Carbohydrate • 401 mg Sodium •
223 mg Calcium • 1 gm Fiber

DIABETIC: 2 Meat • 1 Starch • ½ Vegetable

Micro Pizza Meatloaf

I've always been a big fan of cooking meat in the microwave because you get so much less shrinkage. This particular micro marvel combines some popular pizza toppings with a classic meatloaf preparation, and the end result is sensational! ☻ Serves 6

16 ounces ground 90% lean turkey or beef
6 tablespoons (1½ ounces) dried fine bread crumbs
½ cup finely chopped onion
½ cup finely chopped green bell pepper
½ cup (one 2.5-ounce jar) sliced mushrooms, drained
⅓ cup (1½ ounces) sliced ripe olives
1¾ cups (one 15-ounce can) Hunt's Tomato Sauce☆
2 teaspoons Italian seasoning☆
½ teaspoon Sugar Twin or Sprinkle Sweet
¾ cup (3 ounces) shredded Kraft reduced-fat mozzarella cheese

In a large bowl, combine meat, bread crumbs, onion, green pepper, mushrooms, olives, ½ cup tomato sauce, and 1 teaspoon Italian seasoning. Mix well to combine. Place a small custard cup in center of a deep-dish 9-inch glass pie plate or use a microwave ring mold. Evenly spread meat mixture into plate. Stir remaining 1 teaspoon Italian seasoning and Sugar Twin into remaining 1¼ cups tomato sauce. Spread sauce mixture evenly over meat mixture. Microwave on HIGH (100% power) for 10 minutes. Sprinkle mozzarella cheese evenly over top. Turn dish and continue microwaving on HIGH an additional 8 minutes. Let set for 5 minutes. Cut into 6 servings.

Each serving equals:

HE: 2⅔ Protein • 1⅔ Vegetable • ⅓ Bread • ¼ Fat

201 Calories • 9 gm Fat • 19 gm Protein •
11 gm Carbohydrate • 805 mg Sodium •
117 mg Calcium • 2 gm Fiber

DIABETIC: 2½ Meat • 2 Vegetable

Easy Steak and Mushrooms

Do the cube steaks you prepare too often emerge like pieces of shoe leather? I can do something about that with this simple but delicious recipe! Just think how wonderful it'll be to dine on tender and succulent beef steaks in gravy!   ☻   Serves 4

4 (4-ounce) tenderized lean minute or cube steaks
1 (12-ounce) jar Heinz Fat Free Beef Gravy
1 cup (one 4-ounce jar) sliced mushrooms, drained
⅛ teaspoon black pepper
1 teaspoon dried parsley flakes

In a large skillet sprayed with butter-flavored cooking spray, brown meat for 2 to 3 minutes on each side. In a large bowl, combine beef gravy, mushrooms, black pepper, and parsley flakes. Pour gravy mixture evenly over browned meat. Lower heat, cover, and simmer for 20 minutes or until meat is fork tender. For each serving, place 1 piece of meat on a plate and spoon about ⅓ cup gravy mixture over top.

Each serving equals:

HE: 3 Protein • ½ Vegetable • ¼ Slider •
3 Optional Calories

178 Calories • 6 gm Fat • 26 gm Protein •
5 gm Carbohydrate • 634 mg Sodium •
10 mg Calcium • 1 gm Fiber

DIABETIC: 3 Meat • ½ Vegetable

Fiesta "Steak" with Corn Salsa

The intense flavors of Mexican cooking are often a healthy chef's best friend. In this dish, just a touch of lime juice provides a wonderful tanginess to the meat patties. And instead of spooning salsa from a jar, you'll be creating your very own fresh corn topping that gives this piquant entree some extra sparkle!

☻ Serves 6

> 16 ounces ground 90% turkey or beef
> 6 tablespoons (2¼ ounces) yellow cornmeal
> 1 teaspoon dried parsley flakes
> 2 teaspoons taco seasoning
> 2 teaspoons lime juice☆
> 1 cup (one 8-ounce can) Hunt's Tomato Sauce☆
> 1 cup chunky salsa (mild, medium, or hot)
> 1½ cups frozen or fresh whole-kernel corn
> 1 tablespoon Brown Sugar Twin
> 6 tablespoons Land O Lakes no-fat sour cream

In a large bowl, combine meat, cornmeal, parsley flakes, taco seasoning, 1 teaspoon lime juice, and ¼ cup tomato sauce. Mix well to combine. Using a ⅓-cup measuring cup as a guide, form into 6 patties. Arrange patties in a large skillet sprayed with olive oil–flavored cooking spray. Brown patties for 4 to 5 minutes on each side or until cooked to desired doneness. Meanwhile, in a medium saucepan, combine salsa, corn, remaining ¾ cup tomato sauce, Brown Sugar Twin, and remaining 1 teaspoon lime juice. Cook over medium heat until heated through and patties are done, stirring often. For each serving, place one "steak" on a plate, spoon a full ⅓ cup salsa mixture over meat, and top with 1 tablespoon sour cream.

Each serving equals:

HE: 2 Protein • 1 Bread • 1 Vegetable •
1 Optional Calorie

210 Calories • 6 gm Fat • 16 gm Protein •
23 gm Carbohydrate • 508 mg Sodium •
72 mg Calcium • 3 gm Fiber

DIABETIC: 2 Meat • 1 Starch • 1 Vegetable

BBQ Beef and Potato Hash

This meaty hash is delightfully tangy, so fast to fix, and amazingly filling. Best of all, it delivers lots of protein and fiber for very few calories, and it's low in sodium as well. This will win the hearts of every teenager who tries it, so if you're feeding some growing kids, put this skillet supper on the menu tonight!

☻ Serves 4 (1 cup)

> 1 cup chopped green bell pepper
> ½ cup chopped onion
> 4½ cups (15 ounces) shredded loose-packed frozen potatoes,
>   slightly thawed
> 1 full cup (6 ounces) diced lean cooked roast beef
> ¼ teaspoon black pepper
> ¼ cup Healthy Choice barbeque sauce or any reduced-sodium
>   barbeque sauce

In a large skillet sprayed with butter-flavored cooking spray, sauté green pepper and onion for 5 minutes. Add potatoes. Mix well to combine. Continue cooking for 6 to 10 minutes, or until potatoes are lightly browned, stirring occasionally. Add roast beef and black pepper. Mix lightly to combine. Stir in barbeque sauce. Continue cooking for 5 minutes or until mixture is heated through.

HINTS: 1. Mr. Dell's frozen shredded potatoes are a good choice for this recipe.
            2. If you don't have leftovers, purchase a chunk of lean cooked roast beef from your local deli or use Healthy Choice deli slices.

Each serving equals:

HE: 1½ Protein • ¾ Bread • ¾ Vegetable •
15 Optional Calories

---

168 Calories • 4 gm Fat • 14 gm Protein •
19 gm Carbohydrate • 156 mg Sodium •
12 mg Calcium • 3 gm Fiber

DIABETIC: 1½ Meat • 1 Starch • ½ Vegetable

Gone All Day Stew

I'm so pleased that slow cookers are making a comeback, as mine was a big help to me back when I was going to school, working full-time, and raising my children. I especially like stirring up a delectable meaty stew chock-full of vegetables and potatoes that will smell absolutely scrumptious when you get home from the office.

Serves 6 (1 full cup)

1 (10¾-ounce) can Healthy Request Tomato Soup
¾ cup water
3 tablespoons all-purpose flour
⅛ teaspoon black pepper
1 teaspoon dried parsley flakes
16 ounces lean round steak, cut into 1-inch cubes
1½ cups cut carrots
1 cup coarsely chopped onion
1 cup coarsely cut celery
½ cup (one 2.5-ounce jar) sliced mushrooms, drained
3 cups (15 ounces) diced raw potatoes

In a slow cooker container, combine tomato soup, water, flour, black pepper, and parsley flakes. In a large skillet sprayed with butter-flavored cooking spray, brown meat. Add meat, carrots, onion, celery, mushrooms, and potatoes to mixture in slow cooker. Mix well to combine. Cover and cook on LOW for 6 to 8 hours. Mix well before serving.

Each serving equals:

HE: 2 Protein • 1⅓ Vegetable • ⅔ Bread • ¼ Slider • 10 Optional Calories

212 Calories • 4 gm Fat • 20 gm Protein • 24 gm Carbohydrate • 283 mg Sodium • 39 mg Calcium • 3 gm Fiber

DIABETIC: 2 Meat • 1 Starch • 1 Vegetable

Pepper Pork Tenders with Rice

Pork is definitely one of Cliff's favorite meats, so it's been a real gift to find lean cuts of it in our local supermarkets. This dish is truly luscious, and the chunks of green pepper form a culinary partnership that's bound to please! ☻ Serves 4

1½ cups coarsely chopped green bell pepper
½ cup chopped onion
4 (4-ounce) lean pork tenderloins or cutlets, cut into 16 pieces
½ teaspoon dried minced garlic
1 (10¾-ounce) can Healthy Request Cream of Mushroom Soup
2 cups hot cooked rice

In a large skillet sprayed with butter-flavored cooking spray, sauté green pepper and onion for 5 minutes. Add pork pieces. Mix well to combine. Continue cooking for 5 to 8 minutes, or until pork starts to brown, stirring often. Stir in garlic and mushroom soup. Lower heat, cover, and simmer for 15 minutes. For each serving, place ½ cup rice on a plate and spoon about 1 cup pork mixture over top.

HINT: 1⅓ cups uncooked rice usually cooks to about 2 cups.

Each serving equals:

HE: 3 Protein • 1 Vegetable • 1 Bread • ½ Slider •
1 Optional Calorie

283 Calories • 7 gm Fat • 28 gm Protein •
27 gm Carbohydrate • 379 mg Sodium •
88 mg Calcium • 1 gm Fiber

DIABETIC: 3 Meat • 1½ Starch • ½ Vegetable

Easy Ham Casserole

There's something so appealing about making dinner in the microwave. Maybe it's because you're only dirtying one pot. (You know how I hate to wash dishes. . . .) Maybe it's because you add the ingredients when it makes sense, so nothing turns out over-cooked or undercooked. Or maybe, just maybe, microwaved entrees like this one are mouth-wateringly good!

● Serves 4 (1 full cup)

> 1 cup diced celery
> ½ cup diced onion
> 2 cups (one 16-ounce can) Healthy Request Chicken Broth☆
> ⅔ cup Carnation Nonfat Dry Milk Powder
> 3 tablespoons all-purpose flour
> ¼ cup (¾ ounce) grated Kraft fat-free Parmesan cheese
> ½ cup (one 2.5-ounce jar) sliced mushrooms, drained
> 1½ cups (9 ounces) diced Dubuque 97% fat-free ham or any
>   extra-lean ham
> 2 cups hot cooked spaghetti, rinsed and drained

In an 8-cup glass measuring bowl, combine celery, onion, and 2 tablespoons chicken broth. Microwave on HIGH (100% power) for 2 to 3 minutes or until vegetables are just tender. In a medium bowl, combine dry milk powder, flour, and remaining chicken broth. Mix well using a wire whisk. Blend in Parmesan cheese. Stir broth mixture into vegetables. Cover and microwave on HIGH for 8 to 10 minutes or until mixture thickens, stirring after 4 minutes. Add mushrooms, ham, and spaghetti. Mix well to combine. Re-cover and microwave on HIGH 2 minutes or until mixture is heated through. Let set 5 minutes before serving.

HINT: 1½ cups broken uncooked spaghetti usually cooks to about 2 cups.

Each serving equals:

HE: 1¾ Protein • 1¼ Bread • 1 Vegetable •
½ Skim Milk • 8 Optional Calories

---

263 Calories • 3 gm Fat • 22 gm Protein •
37 gm Carbohydrate • 916 mg Sodium •
178 mg Calcium • 4 gm Fiber

DIABETIC: 2 Meat • 2 Starch • ½ Vegetable
or 2 Meat • 1½ Starch • ½ Vegetable • ½ Skim Milk

Ham Combo Pitas

Ham salad is a Midwest tradition, but the traditional versions are very high in fat and calories. With my magic whisk in hand, however, I created a healthy ham salad as tangy and tasty as it is good for you!   ☻   Serves 6

> 1½ cups (9 ounces) finely diced Dubuque 97% fat-free ham or
>   any extra-lean ham
> 1 cup finely diced celery
> 1 cup shredded carrots
> ½ cup Kraft fat-free mayonnaise
> 1 teaspoon prepared mustard
> 1 teaspoon dried onion flakes
> 1 teaspoon dried parsley flakes
> 2 tablespoons sweet pickle relish
> 3 pita rounds, halved

In a large bowl, combine ham, celery, and carrots. In a small bowl, combine mayonnaise, mustard, onion flakes, parsley flakes, and pickle relish. Add mayonnaise mixture to ham mixture. Mix well to combine. For each sandwich, spoon about ½ cup ham mixture into a pita half. Refrigerate for at least 15 minutes.

HINT: To make opening pita rounds easier, place pita halves on a paper towel and microwave on HIGH for 10 seconds. Remove and gently press open.

Each serving equals:

HE: 1 Bread • 1 Protein • ⅔ Vegetable • ¼ Slider • 3 Optional Calories

134 Calories • 2 gm Fat • 9 gm Protein • 20 gm Carbohydrate • 691 mg Sodium • 42 mg Calcium • 2 gm Fiber

DIABETIC: 1 Starch • 1 Meat • 1 Vegetable

Scalloped Macaroni and Ham

Cheesy. Creamy. Tangy. Even a little sweet (those green peas). Here's an old-timey classic served up quick and easy—and it's sure to please those ravenous family members clamoring for supper!

○ Serves 6

> 1 (10¾-ounce) can Healthy Request Cream of Mushroom Soup
> ½ cup skim milk
> 1½ cups (6 ounces) shredded Kraft reduced-fat Cheddar cheese
> 1 full cup (6 ounces) diced Dubuque 97% fat-free ham or any
>   extra-lean ham
> 1 cup frozen peas, thawed
> 2 cups hot cooked elbow macaroni, rinsed and drained
> ¼ teaspoon black pepper

Preheat oven to 350 degrees. Spray an 8-by-8-inch baking dish with butter-flavored cooking spray. In a large skillet, combine mushroom soup, skim milk, and Cheddar cheese. Cook over medium heat until cheese melts, stirring often. Add ham, peas, macaroni, and black pepper. Mix well to combine. Spread mixture into prepared baking dish. Bake for 30 minutes. Place baking dish on a wire rack and let set for 5 minutes. Divide into 6 servings.

HINTS: 1. Thaw peas by placing in a colander and rinsing under hot water for one minute.
        2. 1⅓ cups uncooked elbow macaroni usually cooks to about 2 cups.

Each serving equals:

HE: 2 Protein • 1 Bread • ¼ Slider •
14 Optional Calories

---

214 Calories • 6 gm Fat • 17 gm Protein •
23 gm Carbohydrate • 690 mg Sodium •
255 mg Calcium • 2 gm Fiber

DIABETIC: 2 Meat • 1½ Starch

Quick Scalloped Potatoes and Ham

Here's a real man-pleasing dish if there ever was one! It certainly appealed to my father-in-law, Cleland, and believe me—if "diet food" passes muster with that man, it has to be good! (You'll notice that I've suggested using canned cooked potatoes in this recipe. If you prefer to use fresh raw potatoes, I suggest slicing them quite thin, and maybe even microwaving them for a few minutes to be certain they're thoroughly cooked.)   ☻   Serves 6

½ cup chopped onion
1 (10¾-ounce) can Healthy Request Cream of Mushroom
   Soup
1 tablespoon all-purpose flour
⅛ teaspoon black pepper
10 ounces (one 16-ounce can) sliced cooked potatoes, rinsed and
   drained
1 full cup (6 ounces) diced Dubuque 97% fat-free ham or any
   extra-lean ham
1 teaspoon dried parsley flakes

Preheat oven to 350 degrees. Spray an 8-by-8-inch baking dish with butter-flavored cooking spray. In a large skillet sprayed with butter-flavored cooking spray, sauté onion for 5 minutes or until tender. Lower heat. Stir in mushroom soup, flour, and black pepper. Layer potatoes and ham in prepared baking dish. Pour sauce over top. Stir to blend. Sprinkle parsley flakes over top. Cover and bake for 20 to 25 minutes. Remove cover and bake an additional 5 to 10 minutes. Place baking dish on a wire rack and let set for 5 minutes. Divide into 6 servings.

Each serving equals:

HE: 1 Bread • 1 Protein • ¼ Vegetable •
4 Optional Calories

130 Calories • 2 gm Fat • 6 gm Protein •
22 gm Carbohydrate • 444 mg Sodium •
41 mg Calcium • 2 gm Fiber

DIABETIC: 1 Starch • 1 Meat

Fettuccine with Ham and Peas

My daughter-in-law Pam loves easy and elegant dishes that are light but still satisfying. This pasta meal is a great example of how you can create a rich and savory dinner in only a couple of steps, but you haven't given anything up in terms of flavor and mouth appeal.

☻ Serves 2 (1 cup)

⅓ cup Carnation Nonfat Dry Milk Powder

½ cup water

½ teaspoon dried minced garlic

½ cup frozen peas, thawed

½ cup (3 ounces) diced Dubuque 97% fat-free ham or any extra-lean ham

1 cup hot cooked fettuccine, rinsed and drained

¼ cup (¾ ounce) grated Kraft fat-free Parmesan cheese

In a small bowl, combine dry milk powder and water. Pour milk mixture into a large skillet sprayed with butter-flavored cooking spray. Add garlic, peas, and ham. Cook over medium heat for 3 minutes or until mixture is hot, but not boiling, stirring often. Add fettuccine and Parmesan cheese. Mix gently to combine. Lower heat and simmer for 5 minutes, or until mixture is heated through, stirring often. Serve at once.

HINTS: 1. Thaw peas by placing in a colander and rinsing under hot water for one minute.
2. ¾ cup broken uncooked fettuccine usually cooks to about 1 cup.

Each serving equals:

HE: 1½ Bread • 1½ Protein • ½ Skim Milk

---

242 Calories • 2 gm Fat • 17 gm Protein •
39 gm Carbohydrate • 584 mg Sodium •
152 mg Calcium • 4 gm Fiber

DIABETIC: 2 Starch • 1½ Meat • ½ Skim Milk

Frank Chop Suey

I'll confess that you probably won't find any traditional Chinese dishes that feature hot dogs, but that's a perfect illustration of why American cooking is truly a melting pot. In this recipe, I've combined our national favorite, the frankfurter, with ingredients common to Chinese food—rice and soy sauce. Add some chopped veggies, simmer, and join in the feast!　❂　Serves 4

1 cup chopped onion

2 cups diced celery

2 cups shredded cabbage

8 ounces Healthy Choice 97% fat-free frankfurters, diced

1 cup hot water

2 tablespoons reduced-sodium soy sauce

2 cups hot cooked rice

In a large skillet sprayed with butter-flavored cooking spray, sauté onion and celery for 5 to 7 minutes or until tender. Add cabbage, frankfurters, and water. Mix well to combine. Lower heat, cover, and simmer for 10 minutes or until liquid is almost absorbed. Stir in soy sauce. For each serving, place ½ cup rice on a plate and spoon 1 full cup of cabbage mixture over top.

HINT:　1⅓ cups uncooked rice usually cooks to about 2 cups.

Each serving equals:

HE: 2½ Vegetable • 1⅓ Protein • 1 Bread

186 Calories • 2 gm Fat • 11 gm Protein •
31 gm Carbohydrate • 887 mg Sodium •
55 mg Calcium • 3 gm Fiber

DIABETIC: 1½ Starch • 1 Vegetable • 1 Meat

Bavarian Pasta-Frankfurter Skillet

Here's another fun, cross-cultural dish that joins German sauerkraut with Italian pasta and those American franks—and the delicious result is a savory skillet supper that celebrates the best of all of us. *Essen! Mangia!* Eat and enjoy! ● Serves 4 (1 full cup)

¼ cup chopped onion

½ cup (one 2.5-ounce jar) sliced mushrooms, drained

1¾ cups (one 14-ounce can) Frank's Bavarian-style sauerkraut, drained

8 ounces (½ package) Healthy Choice 97% fat-free frankfurters, diced

1 (10¾-ounce) can Healthy Request Tomato Soup

2 cups hot cooked rotini pasta, rinsed and drained

1 teaspoon dried parsley flakes

In a large skillet sprayed with butter-flavored cooking spray, sauté onion for 5 minutes or until tender. Stir in mushrooms, sauerkraut, and frankfurters. Add tomato soup, rotini pasta, and parsley flakes. Mix well to combine. Lower heat and simmer for 5 minutes, or until mixture is heated through, stirring occasionally.

HINTS: 1. If you can't find Bavarian sauerkraut, use regular sauerkraut, ½ teaspoon caraway seeds, and 1 teaspoon Brown Sugar Twin.

2. 1½ cups uncooked rotini pasta usually cooks to about 2 cups.

Each serving equals:

HE: 1½ Vegetable • 1⅓ Protein • 1 Bread • ½ Slider • 5 Optional Calories

239 Calories • 3 gm Fat • 13 gm Protein • 40 gm Carbohydrate • 1,571 mg Sodium • 50 mg Calcium • 5 gm Fiber

DIABETIC: 2 Starch • 1½ Meat • 1 Vegetable

Desserts

Baked Pears with Apricot Filling

As much as I enjoy snacking on fresh fruit, I often find much more "mouth satisfaction" in a baked version of that fruit instead. Here's a perfect example of how to take something already quite delicious—a ripe pear—and by baking it and topping it, you make it something truly spectacular!   ☻   Serves 4 (2 halves)

> 4 medium-sized cored, unpeeled, and halved ripe pears
> 2 tablespoons apricot spreadable fruit
> 6 tablespoons purchased graham cracker crumbs or 6 (2½-inch)
>   graham crackers made into crumbs
> 2 tablespoons (½ ounce) chopped pecans
> 1 tablespoon Sugar Twin or Sprinkle Sweet

Place pear halves in an 8-by-8-inch baking dish, cut side up. Cover and microwave on HIGH (100% power) for 2 minutes. Place a full teaspoon spreadable fruit in center of each pear. In a small bowl, combine graham cracker crumbs, pecans, and Sugar Twin. Evenly sprinkle crumb mixture over top. Re-cover and continue to microwave on HIGH for 2 to 4 minutes or until pears are soft. Divide into 4 servings. Serve warm.

Each serving equals:

HE: 1½ Fruit • ½ Bread • ½ Fat • 1 Optional Calorie

192 Calories • 4 gm Fat • 2 gm Protein •
37 gm Carbohydrate • 76 mg Sodium •
62 mg Calcium • 4 gm Fiber

DIABETIC: 1½ Fruit • ½ Starch • ½ Fat

Lemon Mousse

Is there anything more lush and creamy, tart and sweet, than this pretty confection? By layering the flavor of lemon (with the Diet Dew), this recipe intensifies the pleasure—and soothes the soul!

◐ Serves 6

> 1 (4-serving) package JELL-O sugar-free instant vanilla pudding mix
> 1 (4-serving) package JELL-O sugar-free lemon gelatin
> ⅔ cup Carnation Nonfat Dry Milk Powder
> 1 cup Diet Mountain Dew
> ¾ cup Yoplait plain fat-free yogurt
> ¾ cup Cool Whip Lite

In a large bowl, combine dry pudding mix, dry gelatin, and dry milk powder. Add Diet Mountain Dew. Mix well using a wire whisk. Blend in yogurt and Cool Whip Lite. Spoon mixture into 6 dessert dishes. Refrigerate for at least 15 minutes.

Each serving equals:

HE: ½ Skim Milk • ½ Slider • 3 Optional Calories

81 Calories • 1 gm Fat • 5 gm Protein •
13 gm Carbohydrate • 323 mg Sodium •
148 mg Calcium • 0 gm Fiber

DIABETIC: ½ Skim Milk • ½ Starch
or 1 Starch/Carbohydrate

Pineapple Blueberry Custard Cups

In most parts of the country, the season for affordable fresh blueberries isn't long, so join me in seizing the moment and stirring up this tasty dessert. This looks irresistible, so surrender to temptation—and enjoy! Serves 4

1½ cups fresh blueberries☆
1 (4-serving) package JELL-O sugar-free vanilla cook-and-serve pudding mix
⅔ cup Carnation Nonfat Dry Milk Powder
1 cup water
1 cup (one 8-ounce can) crushed pineapple, packed in fruit juice, undrained
1 teaspoon vanilla extract
⅛ teaspoon ground nutmeg
¼ cup Cool Whip Lite

Reserve ¼ cup blueberries. Evenly divide remaining 1¼ cups blueberries into 4 dessert dishes. In a medium saucepan, combine dry pudding mix, dry milk powder, water, and undrained pineapple. Cook over medium heat until mixture thickens and starts to boil, stirring constantly. Remove from heat. Stir in vanilla extract and nutmeg. Evenly spoon hot mixture over blueberries. Refrigerate for at least 1 hour. When serving, top each with 1 tablespoon Cool Whip Lite and 1 tablespoon reserved blueberries.

Each serving equals:

HE: 1 Fruit • ½ Skim Milk • ¼ Slider • 10 Optional Calories

---

149 Calories • 1 gm Fat • 5 gm Protein • 30 gm Carbohydrate • 395 mg Sodium • 150 mg Calcium • 2 gm Fiber

---

DIABETIC: 1 Fruit • ½ Skim Milk • ½ Starch *or* 2 Starch/Carbohydrate

Chocolate-Covered Cherry Pudding

Remember the sensation of biting into a chocolate-covered cherry? There's the rich taste of chocolate, and some impossibly sweet liquid, along with the creamy coating of the cherry in the center. I closed my eyes and recalled all those fantastic flavors when I created this special pudding, and I think I got pretty close! My father, Jerome McAndrews, loved chocolate-covered cherries, so this recipe would have made him smile with pleasure!

☻ Serves 6

> 1 (4-serving) package JELL-O sugar-free instant chocolate fudge
>   pudding mix
> ⅔ cup Carnation Nonfat Dry Milk Powder
> 2 cups (one 16-ounce can) tart red cherries, packed in water,
>   drained, and ½ cup liquid reserved
> ½ cup water
> ¾ cup Cool Whip Free
> ¾ cup Yoplait plain fat-free yogurt
> 1 teaspoon brandy extract

In a large bowl, combine dry pudding mix and dry milk powder. Add reserved cherry liquid and water. Mix well using a wire whisk. Blend in Cool Whip Free, yogurt, and brandy extract. Add cherries. Mix gently to combine. Evenly spoon mixture into 6 dessert dishes. Refrigerate for at least 15 minutes.

Each serving equals:

HE: ⅔ Fruit • ½ Skim Milk • ½ Slider • 3 Optional Calories

109 Calories • 1 gm Fat • 5 gm Protein • 20 gm Carbohydrate • 288 mg Sodium • 157 mg Calcium • 1 gm Fiber

DIABETIC: 1 Fruit • ½ Skim Milk
or 1 Starch/Carbohydrate • ½ Skim Milk

Old-Fashioned Tapioca Pudding

Sometimes, when we gobble down our desserts, we're reliving sweet memories of childhood. For Cliff, the most important dessert memory he has is of tapioca pudding prepared the old-fashioned way. Well, I rarely take the time to stir up the long-cooking version, but he told me that this recipe comes amazingly close to that great old taste! ❤ Serves 4

> 3 tablespoons quick tapioca
> 1 (4-serving) package JELL-O sugar-free vanilla cook-and-serve pudding mix
> 2 tablespoons Sugar Twin or Sprinkle Sweet
> 2 cups skim milk
> ½ cup water
> ½ teaspoon vanilla extract
> ¼ cup Cool Whip Lite

In a medium saucepan, combine tapioca, dry pudding mix, Sugar Twin, skim milk, and water. Mix well to combine. Let set for 5 minutes. Cook over medium heat, until mixture thickens and starts to boil, stirring often. Remove from heat. Stir in vanilla extract. Evenly spoon mixture into 4 dessert dishes. Refrigerate for at least 15 minutes. When serving, top each with 1 tablespoon Cool Whip Lite.

Each serving equals:

HE: ½ Skim Milk • ½ Slider • 16 Optional Calories

97 Calories • 1 gm Fat • 4 gm Protein •
18 gm Carbohydrate • 178 mg Sodium •
152 mg Calcium • 0 gm Fiber

DIABETIC: ½ Skim Milk • ½ Starch
or 1 Starch/Carbohydrate

Mocha Crunch Pudding

Since I'm not really a fan of coffee-flavored desserts, I asked for lots of other opinions when I was testing this recipe. (I also featured it at our Taste-Testing Buffet, where it received A+ ratings across the board!) Everyone agreed this was downright scrumptious, from the rich-tasting pudding to the crunchy crumbs and chips!

☻ Serves 6

1 (4-serving) package JELL-O sugar-free instant chocolate fudge
    pudding mix
⅔ cup Carnation Nonfat Dry Milk Powder
1¼ cups cold coffee
¾ cup Yoplait plain fat-free yogurt
¾ cup Cool Whip Lite☆
9 (2½-inch) chocolate graham crackers made into crumbs
1 tablespoon (¼ ounce) mini chocolate chips

In a large bowl, combine dry pudding mix, dry milk powder, and cold coffee. Mix well using a wire whisk. Blend in yogurt and ¼ cup Cool Whip Lite. Add graham cracker crumbs. Mix gently to combine. Evenly spoon mixture into 6 dessert dishes. Top each with 1 tablespoon Cool Whip Lite and ½ teaspoon chocolate chips. Refrigerate for at least 5 minutes.

HINT: A self-seal sandwich bag works great for crushing graham crackers.

Each serving equals:

HE: ½ Skim Milk • ½ Bread • ½ Slider •
10 Optional Calories

---

114 Calories • 2 gm Fat • 5 gm Protein •
19 gm Carbohydrate • 317 mg Sodium •
150 mg Calcium • 0 gm Fiber

DIABETIC: 1 Starch • ½ Skim Milk

Maple-Raisin-Pecan Pudding Treats

Whenever I make butterscotch pudding desserts, I think about Becky Ann, my daughter, who always adored them. And even though she lives so far away from DeWitt, when I stirred up this sweet and crunchy blend, it felt almost as if she were in the kitchen with me! This one's for you, Becky.   ☻   Serves 4

1 (4-serving) package JELL-O sugar-free instant butterscotch
    pudding mix
2/3 cup Carnation Nonfat Dry Milk Powder
1¼ cups water
½ cup Cary's Sugar Free Maple Syrup
½ cup Cool Whip Lite☆
½ cup raisins
1 tablespoon (¼ ounce) chopped pecans

In a large bowl, combine dry pudding mix and dry milk powder. Add water and maple syrup. Mix well using a wire whisk. Blend in ¼ cup Cool Whip Lite and raisins. Evenly spoon mixture into 4 dessert dishes. Top each with 1 tablespoon Cool Whip Lite and ¾ teaspoon chopped pecans.

HINT: To plump up raisins without "cooking," place in a glass measuring cup and microwave on HIGH for 15 seconds.

Each serving equals:

HE: 1 Fruit • ½ Skim Milk • ¼ Fat • ¾ Slider •
5 Optional Calories

170 Calories • 2 gm Fat • 5 gm Protein •
33 gm Carbohydrate • 471 mg Sodium •
147 mg Calcium • 1 gm Fiber

DIABETIC: 1 Fruit • 1 Starch • ½ Skim Milk
or 2 Starch/Carbohydrate

White Chocolate Rice Pudding

There are two groups of people in the world: (I'm writing this with a smile . . .) those who like ice cream and pudding with "things" in them—nuts, fruit, candy, et cetera; and those who like theirs perfectly smooth. I created this inviting combo for the first group, who will cheer each nibble of pecan or chocolate chip they find. (I also created it for Cliff, who never met a rice pudding he didn't like. . . .)

◐ Serves 4

1 (4-serving) package JELL-O sugar-free instant white chocolate pudding mix
⅔ cup Carnation Nonfat Dry Milk Powder
1½ cups water
½ cup Cool Whip Free
1½ cups cold cooked rice
2 tablespoons (½ ounce) mini chocolate chips
2 tablespoons (½ ounce) chopped pecans

In a large bowl, combine dry pudding mix, dry milk powder, and water. Mix well using a wire whisk. Blend in Cool Whip Free. Add rice, chocolate chips, and pecans. Mix gently to combine. Evenly spoon mixture into 4 dessert dishes. Refrigerate for at least 15 minutes.

HINT: 1 cup uncooked rice usually cooks to about 1½ cups.

Each serving equals:

HE: ¾ Bread • ½ Skim Milk • ½ Fat • ¾ Slider • 9 Optional Calories

168 Calories • 4 gm Fat • 5 gm Protein • 28 gm Carbohydrate • 394 mg Sodium • 146 mg Calcium • 1 gm Fiber

DIABETIC: 1½ Starch/Carbohydrate • ½ Skim Milk • ½ Fat or 2 Starch/Carbohydrate • ½ Skim Milk

Orange Sunshine Rice Pudding

Rice pudding is such a wonderfully cozy and old-fashioned dessert, but it also appeals to the current generation of kids. My own grandchildren particularly enjoyed this version, which turns a lovely pale orange when the orange juice and oranges are mixed in. If ever a dessert tasted like a summer sunrise, this would be it!

◐ Serves 4

> 1 (4-serving) package JELL-O sugar-free instant vanilla pudding mix
> ⅔ cup Carnation Nonfat Dry Milk Powder
> ½ cup unsweetened orange juice
> ½ cup cold water
> ½ cup Cool Whip Free
> 1½ cups cold cooked rice
> 1 cup (one 11-ounce can) mandarin oranges, rinsed and drained

In a large bowl, combine dry pudding mix, dry milk powder, orange juice, and water. Mix well using a wire whisk. Blend in Cool Whip Free. Add rice and mandarin oranges. Mix gently to combine. Evenly spoon mixture into 4 dessert dishes. Refrigerate for at least 15 minutes.

HINT: 1 cup uncooked rice usually cooks to about 1½ cups.

Each serving equals:

HE: ¾ Fruit • ¾ Bread • ½ Skim Milk • ½ Slider • 5 Optional Calories

---

174 Calories • 1 gm Fat • 6 gm Protein • 35 gm Carbohydrate • 397 mg Sodium • 152 mg Calcium • 1 gm Fiber

---

DIABETIC: 1 Starch • ½ Fruit • ½ Skim Milk *or* 2 Starch/Carbohydrate

New Orleans Bread Pudding

I'm the true bread pudding fan in our house, and it's just about the only dessert I'll order when Cliff and I dine out during my book tours. This dish was inspired by our visit to the "Big Easy," where people love to eat just as much as they love their music. Is there anything better than a warm piece of bread pudding, with a rich sauce poured over it? *Mmm-mmm . . .*   ☻   Serves 6

> 2 (4-serving) packages JELL-O sugar-free vanilla cook-and-serve
>   pudding mix☆
> 4 cups skim milk☆
> 1 teaspoon coconut extract
> ½ teaspoon ground nutmeg
> 8 slices reduced-calorie French or white bread, torn into pieces
> ½ cup raisins
> 2 tablespoons flaked coconut
> 2 tablespoons (½ ounce) chopped pecans
> 1 teaspoon rum extract
> 2 teaspoons reduced-calorie margarine

Preheat oven to 350 degrees. Spray an 8-by-8-inch baking dish with butter-flavored cooking spray. In a large skillet, combine 1 package dry pudding mix and 2½ cups skim milk. Cook over medium heat until mixture starts to boil, stirring constantly. Remove from heat. Stir in coconut extract and nutmeg. Add bread pieces, raisins, coconut, and pecans. Mix gently to combine. Pour mixture into prepared baking dish. Bake for 30 to 35 minutes. Place baking dish on a wire rack while preparing sauce. In a medium saucepan, combine remaining dry pudding mix and remaining 1½ cups skim milk. Cook over medium heat until mixture thickens and starts to boil, stirring constantly. Remove from heat. Stir in rum extract and margarine. Cut warm bread pudding into 6 servings. For each serving, place 1 piece of bread pudding on a serving plate and spoon about ¼ cup warm rum sauce over top.

Each serving equals:

HE: ⅔ Skim Milk • ⅔ Bread • ⅔ Fruit • ½ Fat •
¼ Slider • 12 Optional Calories

211 Calories • 3 gm Fat • 10 gm Protein •
36 gm Carbohydrate • 652 mg Sodium •
231 mg Calcium • 1 gm Fiber

DIABETIC: 1 Skim Milk • 1 Fruit • ½ Starch • ½ Fat

James's Cherry-Pineapple Dessert

When he peeked into my refrigerator and spotted this pretty fruit dessert, it didn't take long for my son James to cut a piece and gobble it down! (He really LOVES cherries!) The pineapple and cherries go beautifully together, and the delicate touch of almond makes a good dessert a great one. ○ Serves 8

> 12 (2½-inch) graham cracker squares☆
> 1 (4-serving) package JELL-O sugar-free instant vanilla pudding mix
> ⅔ cup Carnation Nonfat Dry Milk Powder
> 1 cup water
> 1 cup Cool Whip Lite☆
> 1 (4-serving) package JELL-O sugar-free vanilla cook-and-serve pudding mix
> 1 (4-serving) package JELL-O sugar-free cherry gelatin
> 1 cup (one 8-ounce can) crushed pineapple, packed in fruit juice, undrained
> 2 cups (one 16-ounce can) tart red cherries, packed in water, undrained
> 1 teaspoon almond extract

Evenly arrange 9 graham crackers in a 9-by-9-inch cake pan. In a medium bowl, combine dry instant vanilla pudding mix, dry milk powder, and water. Mix well using a wire whisk. Blend in ½ cup Cool Whip Lite. Spread pudding mixture evenly over graham crackers. Refrigerate. Meanwhile, in a medium saucepan, combine dry vanilla cook-and-serve pudding mix, dry gelatin, and undrained pineapple. Stir in undrained cherries. Cook over medium heat until mixture thickens and starts to boil, stirring often, being careful not to crush cherries. Remove from heat. Stir in almond extract. Place pan on a wire rack and allow to cool for 15 minutes. Evenly spoon cherry mixture over pudding layer. Crush

remaining 3 graham crackers and evenly sprinkle crumbs over top.
Cover and refrigerate for at least 2 hours. Cut into 8 servings. When
serving, top each piece with 1 tablespoon Cool Whip Lite.

HINT: A self-seal sandwich bag works great for crushing graham
   crackers.

Each serving equals:

HE: ¾ Fruit • ½ Bread • ¼ Skim Milk • ½ Slider •
8 Optional Calories

---

154 Calories • 2 gm Fat • 4 gm Protein •
30 gm Carbohydrate • 367 mg Sodium •
80 mg Calcium • 1 gm Fiber

DIABETIC: 1 Fruit • 1 Starch/Carbohydrate
or 2 Starch/Carbohydrate

Chocolate Cherry Dessert

If you've ever tasted Black Forest Cake, you know that the combo of chocolate and cherries is utterly luscious! Well, here's my take on this European favorite that's become an American tradition. The mayonnaise provides a little baking magic and produces a wonderfully moist cake. ☺ Serves 12

 1 (4-serving) package JELL-O sugar-free vanilla cook-and-serve pudding mix
 1 (4-serving) package JELL-O sugar-free cherry gelatin
 2 cups (one 16-ounce can) tart red cherries, packed in water, undrained
 2¾ cups water☆
 2 teaspoons almond extract☆
 1½ cups all-purpose flour
 ¼ cup unsweetened cocoa
 1 teaspoon baking soda
 ½ cup Sugar Twin or Sprinkle Sweet
 ¾ cup Kraft fat-free mayonnaise
 1 (4-serving) package JELL-O sugar-free instant chocolate fudge pudding mix
 1 cup Carnation Nonfat Dry Milk Powder
 ½ cup Cool Whip Lite
 2 tablespoons (½ ounce) chopped almonds

Preheat oven to 350 degrees. Spray a 9-by-9-inch cake pan with butter-flavored cooking spray. In a medium saucepan, combine dry cook-and-serve pudding mix, dry gelatin, undrained cherries, and ¾ cup water. Cook over medium heat until mixture thickens and starts to boil, stirring constantly. Remove from heat. Stir in 1 teaspoon almond extract. Place pan on a wire rack and allow to cool. Meanwhile, in a large bowl, combine flour, cocoa, baking soda, and Sugar Twin. Add mayonnaise, ¾ cup water, and ½ teaspoon almond extract. Mix well to combine. Pour mixture into prepared cake pan. Bake for 18 to 22 minutes or until toothpick inserted in center comes out clean. Do not overbake. Place cake pan on a wire rack and allow to cool for 5 minutes. Spread cooled cherry mixture evenly over slightly cooled cake. Continue to cool 30 minutes. In a medium bowl, combine dry instant pudding mix, dry milk powder, and remaining 1¼ cups water. Mix well using a wire whisk. Blend in Cool Whip Lite and remaining ½ teaspoon almond extract. Spread pudding mixture evenly over cherry layer. Sprinkle chopped almonds evenly over top. Refrigerate for at least 30 minutes. Cut into 12 servings.

Each serving equals:

HE: ⅔ Bread • ⅓ Fruit • ¼ Skim Milk • ½ Slider • 19 Optional Calories

227 Calories • 3 gm Fat • 8 gm Protein • 42 gm Carbohydrate • 660 mg Sodium • 82 mg Calcium • 2 gm Fiber

DIABETIC: 2 Starch/Carbohydrate • ½ Fruit

Layered Rhubarb Cream Dessert

If Iowa had a state fruit, it would probably be rhubarb! Once the first rhubarb of the season appears at our markets and farm stands, it's probably only a few hours before the rhubarb pies start emerging from our ovens! This creamy dessert makes a deserving star of this sweet, tart treasure.   ☯   Serves 8

12 (2½-inch) graham cracker squares☆
1 (4-serving) package JELL-O sugar-free vanilla cook-and-serve
    pudding mix
1 (4-serving) package JELL-O sugar-free strawberry gelatin
2 cups water☆
2 cups finely chopped rhubarb
1 (4-serving) JELL-O sugar-free instant vanilla pudding mix
⅔ cup Carnation Nonfat Dry Milk Powder
½ cup Cool Whip Lite

Evenly arrange 9 graham crackers in a 9-by-9-inch cake pan. In a large saucepan, combine dry cook-and-serve pudding mix, dry gelatin, and 1 cup water. Stir in rhubarb. Cook over medium heat until rhubarb softens and mixture starts to boil, stirring constantly. Remove from heat. Evenly spoon rhubarb mixture over graham crackers. Refrigerate for 30 minutes. In a medium bowl, combine dry instant pudding mix, dry milk powder, and remaining 1 cup water. Mix well using a wire whisk. Blend in Cool Whip Lite. Evenly spread pudding mixture over rhubarb layer. Crush remaining 3 graham crackers and evenly sprinkle crumbs over top. Cover and refrigerate for at least 2 hours. Cut into 8 servings.

HINT: A self-seal sandwich bag works great for crushing graham
    crackers.

Each serving equals:

HE: ½ Bread • ½ Vegetable • ¼ Slider •
18 Optional Calories

106 Calories • 2 gm Fat • 3 gm Protein •
19 gm Carbohydrate • 364 mg Sodium •
95 mg Calcium • 1 gm Fiber

DIABETIC: 1 Starch/Carbohydrate

Peaches and Strawberry Shortcakes with Orange Cream Topping

My other most favorite dessert (besides bread pudding) is fresh strawberry shortcake, so I enjoy creating (and testing!) recipes that feature that perfect red gem of fruits! This time, though, I decided to introduce some luscious fresh peaches into the mix—as well as a creamy sauce on top. Taste it, and I bet you'll echo my reaction: It's a real show-stopper! ❤ Serves 4

> ¾ cup Bisquick Reduced Fat Baking Mix
> ⅓ cup Carnation Nonfat Dry Milk Powder
> ½ cup Sugar Twin or Sprinkle Sweet☆
> 2 tablespoons Kraft fat-free mayonnaise
> ⅓ cup water
> 1 teaspoon vanilla extract
> 2½ cups sliced fresh strawberries☆
> 1 cup (2 medium) peeled and sliced fresh peaches
> ½ cup (4 ounces) Philadelphia fat-free cream cheese
> ¼ cup unsweetened orange juice
> ½ cup Cool Whip Lite

Preheat oven to 415 degrees. Spray a baking sheet with butter-flavored cooking spray. In a medium bowl, combine baking mix, dry milk powder, and ¼ cup Sugar Twin. Add mayonnaise, water, and vanilla extract. Mix well to combine. Drop by spoonfuls onto prepared baking sheet to form 4 shortcakes. Bake for 8 to 10 minutes or until golden brown. Place baking sheet on a wire rack and allow to cool. Meanwhile, in a medium bowl, mash 1 cup strawberries with a fork or potato masher. Stir in remaining ¼ cup Sugar Twin. Add remaining 1½ cups strawberries and peaches. Mix gently to combine. Cover and refrigerate. Meanwhile, in a small bowl, stir cream cheese with a spoon until soft. Add orange juice and Cool Whip Lite. Mix gently to combine. For each serving, place 1 shortcake in a dessert dish, spoon about a full ½ cup strawberry mixture over shortcake, and top with ¼ cup topping mixture.

Each serving equals:

HE: 1¼ Fruit • 1 Bread • ½ Protein • ¼ Skim Milk • ¼ Slider • 15 Optional Calories

---

215 Calories • 3 gm Fat • 9 gm Protein •
38 gm Carbohydrate • 531 mg Sodium •
105 mg Calcium • 3 gm Fiber

DIABETIC: 1½ Starch/Carbohydrate • 1 Fruit • ½ Meat

Apple Harvest Cobbler

You know how it feels to come home from picking apples in an orchard and be faced with a huge pile of fruit? You think, well, I'll make applesauce. I'll make pie. I'll bake bread. And well you might. But first, why not stir up this tasty cobbler that is just ideal for brunch on a cool autumn morning? It's a winner!

○ Serves 6

> 1 (4-serving) package JELL-O sugar-free vanilla cook-and-serve
>   pudding mix
> 1 teaspoon apple pie spice
> 1 tablespoon Brown Sugar Twin
> 1 cup unsweetened apple juice
> 2 cups (4 small) cored, unpeeled, and sliced cooking
>   apples
> ¼ cup (1 ounce) chopped walnuts
> 1 (7.5-ounce) can Pillsbury refrigerated buttermilk
>   biscuits
> 2 tablespoons Sugar Twin or Sprinkle Sweet

Preheat oven to 350 degrees. Spray an 8-by-8-inch baking dish with butter-flavored cooking spray. In a large saucepan, combine dry pudding mix, apple pie spice, Brown Sugar Twin, and apple juice. Add apples. Mix well to combine. Cook over medium heat until mixture thickens and starts to boil, stirring often. Stir in walnuts. Pour mixture into prepared baking dish. Separate biscuits and cut each into 4 pieces. Evenly sprinkle biscuit pieces over top. Lightly spray tops with butter-flavored cooking spray. Sprinkle Sugar Twin evenly over top. Bake for 20 to 25 minutes or until top is golden brown. Place baking dish on a wire rack and allow to cool. Cut into 6 servings.

Each serving equals:

HE: 1¼ Bread • 1 Fruit • ⅓ Fat • ¼ Slider •
6 Optional Calories

---

176 Calories • 4 gm Fat • 3 gm Protein •
32 gm Carbohydrate • 382 mg Sodium •
10 mg Calcium • 3 gm Fiber

DIABETIC: 1 Starch • 1 Fruit • ½ Fat
or 2 Starch/Carbohydrate • ½ Fat

Praline Apple Dessert

Delicious decadence—how else to describe pecan pralines, that sweet Louisiana confection that's just about pure sugar! I choose not to indulge in the "real thing," but this delectable apple dessert delivers more than enough of that taste sensation to satisfy me. I bet it'll please you just as much! ☻ Serves 6

1 (4-serving) package JELL-O sugar-free instant butterscotch pudding mix
⅓ cup Carnation Nonfat Dry Milk Powder
¾ cup Yoplait plain fat-free yogurt
½ cup unsweetened apple juice
¾ cup Cool Whip Lite☆
½ teaspoon apple pie spice
¼ cup (1 ounce) chopped pecans
1½ cups (3 small) cored, unpeeled, and chopped Red Delicious apples
6 tablespoons purchased graham cracker crumbs or 6 (2½-inch) graham crackers made into crumbs
2 tablespoons caramel syrup

In a large bowl, combine dry pudding mix, dry milk powder, yogurt, and apple juice. Mix well using a wire whisk. Blend in ¼ cup Cool Whip Lite, apple pie spice, and pecans. Add apples and graham cracker crumbs. Mix gently to combine. Spoon mixture evenly into 6 dessert dishes. Garnish each with 1 tablespoon Cool Whip Lite and drizzle 1 teaspoon caramel syrup over top. Refrigerate for at least 15 minutes.

Each serving equals:

HE: ⅔ Fat • ½ Fruit • ⅓ Skim Milk • ⅓ Bread • ¼ Slider • 17 Optional Calories

173 Calories • 5 gm Fat • 4 gm Protein • 28 gm Carbohydrate • 338 mg Sodium • 113 mg Calcium • 1 gm Fiber

DIABETIC: 1 Fat • 1 Starch/Carbohydrate • ½ Fruit *or* 1½ Starch/Carbohydrate • 1 Fat

Anna's Poofy Lemon Chiffon Pie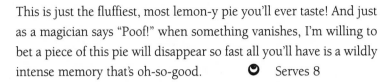

This is just the fluffiest, most lemon-y pie you'll ever taste! And just as a magician says "Poof!" when something vanishes, I'm willing to bet a piece of this pie will disappear so fast all you'll have is a wildly intense memory that's oh-so-good.   ☻   Serves 8

1 cup Diet Mountain Dew or water
¼ of a lemon, with skin and seeds, cut into chunks
1 (4-serving) package JELL-O sugar-free instant vanilla pudding
    mix
1 tub Crystal Light Lemonade Mix
⅔ cup Carnation Nonfat Dry Milk Powder
1½ cups Yoplait plain fat-free yogurt
1 cup Cool Whip Lite☆
1 (6-ounce) Keebler shortbread piecrust

In a blender container, combine Diet Mountain Dew and lemon chunks. Cover and process on BLEND for 60 seconds or until lemon pieces almost disappear. Set aside. In a large bowl, combine dry pudding mix, dry lemonade mix, and dry milk powder. Add Diet Mountain Dew mixture and yogurt. Mix well using a wire whisk. Blend in ¼ cup Cool Whip Lite. Spread pudding mixture into piecrust. Refrigerate for 5 minutes. Drop remaining Cool Whip Lite by tablespoonfuls to form 8 mounds. Refrigerate for at least 2 hours. Cut into 8 servings.

Each serving equals:

HE: ½ Bread • ½ Skim Milk • 1 Slider •
1 Optional Calorie

182 Calories • 6 gm Fat • 5 gm Protein •
27 gm Carbohydrate • 352 mg Sodium •
154 mg Calcium • 1 gm Fiber

DIABETIC: 1½ Starch/Carbohydrate • 1 Fat •
½ Skim Milk

Chunky Chocolate Cream Pie

Just because you've chosen a healthy lifestyle over your old favorite nutty-fruity chocolate candy doesn't mean never savoring those outrageously good flavors again. Far from it, in fact. Here's a pie that's almost like a candy bar in a piecrust! *Mmm-mmm!*

❂ Serves 8

> 1 (4-serving) package JELL-O sugar-free instant chocolate
>   pudding mix
> ⅔ cup Carnation Nonfat Dry Milk Powder
> 1¼ cups water
> 1 teaspoon vanilla extract
> 1 cup Cool Whip Free☆
> 1 cup raisins
> 1 tablespoon (¼ ounce) mini chocolate chips
> 2 tablespoons (½ ounce) chopped pecans
> 1 (6-ounce) Keebler chocolate piecrust
> 1 teaspoon coconut extract
> 2 tablespoons flaked coconut

In a large bowl, combine dry pudding mix, dry milk powder, and water. Mix well using a wire whisk. Blend in vanilla extract and ¼ cup Cool Whip Free. Gently fold in raisins, chocolate chips, and pecans. Spread mixture evenly into piecrust. Refrigerate for 30 minutes. In a small bowl, combine remaining ¾ cup Cool Whip Free and coconut extract. Spread mixture evenly over set pudding. Evenly sprinkle coconut over top. Refrigerate for at least 2 hours. Cut into 8 servings.

HINT: To plump up raisins without "cooking," place in a glass measuring cup and microwave on HIGH for 20 seconds.

Each serving equals:

HE: 1 Fruit • ½ Bread • ¼ Skim Milk • ¼ Fat •
1 Slider • 7 Optional Calories

243 Calories • 7 gm Fat • 4 gm Protein •
41 gm Carbohydrate • 306 mg Sodium •
79 mg Calcium • 1 gm Fiber

DIABETIC: 1½ Starch/Carbohydrate • 1 Fruit • 1 Fat

Double Decker Chocolate-Cream Pie

If one layer of chocolate cream is luscious, you just can't go wrong with two! Add to that a chocolate crust and a few chocolate chips, and you've got a prize-winning dessert that's perfect for any celebration.   ☻   Serves 8

1 (4-serving) package JELL-O sugar-free instant chocolate fudge
    pudding mix
1⅓ cups Carnation Nonfat Dry Milk Powder☆
2¼ cups water☆
1 (6-ounce) Keebler chocolate piecrust
1 (4-serving) package JELL-O sugar-free instant white chocolate
    pudding mix
½ cup Cool Whip Free
1 (2½-inch) chocolate graham cracker square made into fine
    crumbs
1 tablespoon (¼ ounce) mini chocolate chips

In a large bowl, combine dry chocolate fudge pudding mix, ⅔ cup dry milk powder, and 1¼ cups water. Mix well using a wire whisk. Pour mixture evenly into piecrust. Refrigerate while preparing topping. In another large bowl, combine dry white chocolate pudding mix, remaining ⅔ cup dry milk powder, and remaining 1 cup water. Mix well using a wire whisk. Blend in Cool Whip Free. Evenly spread topping mixture over chocolate fudge layer. Sprinkle graham cracker crumbs and chocolate chips evenly over top. Refrigerate for at least 1 hour. Cut into 8 servings.

HINT: A self-seal sandwich bag works great for crushing graham crackers.

Each serving equals:

HE: ½ Bread • ½ Skim Milk • 1 Slider •
19 Optional Calories

---

194 Calories • 6 gm Fat • 5 gm Protein •
30 gm Carbohydrate • 497 mg Sodium •
139 mg Calcium • 1 gm Fiber

DIABETIC: 1½ Starch • 1 Fat • ½ Skim Milk

Valley State Bank Banana Cream Pie

I created this pie for the grand opening of a new bank in Bettendorf, Iowa. It was inspired by the favorite flavors of the bank president, but I'll bet someone you know will relish it just as much!

● Serves 8

> 2 cups (2 medium) diced bananas
> 1 (6-ounce) Keebler shortbread piecrust
> 1 (4-serving) package JELL-O sugar-free instant banana cream pudding mix
> ⅔ cup Carnation Nonfat Dry Milk Powder
> 1¼ cups water
> 1 teaspoon almond extract☆
> 1 cup Cool Whip Free☆
> 2 tablespoons (½ ounce) chopped almonds
> 4 maraschino cherries, halved

Layer bananas in bottom of piecrust. In a large bowl, combine dry pudding mix, dry milk powder, and water. Mix well using a wire whisk. Blend in ½ teaspoon almond extract and ¼ cup Cool Whip Free. Spread pudding mixture evenly over bananas. Refrigerate while preparing topping. In a small bowl, combine remaining ¾ cup Cool Whip Free and remaining ½ teaspoon almond extract. Spread topping mixture evenly over set filling. Evenly sprinkle almonds over top and garnish with cherry halves. Refrigerate for at least 1 hour. Cut into 8 servings.

HINT: To prevent bananas from turning brown, mix with 1 teaspoon lemon juice or sprinkle with Fruit Fresh.

Each serving equals:

HE: ½ Bread • ½ Fruit • ¼ Skim Milk • 1 Slider • 9 Optional Calories

---

207 Calories • 7 gm Fat • 4 gm Protein • 32 gm Carbohydrate • 321 mg Sodium • 77 mg Calcium • 1 gm Fiber

---

DIABETIC: 1½ Starch/Carbohydrate • 1 Fat • ½ Fruit

Rhubarb-Banana Cream Pie

What a festive melange of flavors in this rich and creamy dessert! You usually find rhubarb coupled with strawberries, but it's equally luscious when holding hands with banana. If you've never tried rhubarb (are there any of you left?), give this special pie a chance to win your heart. ☺ Serves 8

1 cup (1 medium) diced banana
1 (6-ounce) Keebler graham cracker piecrust
1 (4-serving) package JELL-O sugar-free vanilla cook-and-serve
    pudding mix
1 (4-serving) package JELL-O sugar-free strawberry gelatin
1 cup water
2 cups finely chopped rhubarb
1 (8-ounce) package Philadelphia fat-free cream cheese
2 tablespoons graham cracker crumbs or 2 (2½-inch) graham
    cracker squares made into crumbs
½ cup Cool Whip Lite

Layer banana in bottom of piecrust. In a large saucepan, combine dry pudding mix, dry gelatin, and water. Stir in rhubarb. Cook over medium heat, until rhubarb softens and mixture thickens, stirring constantly. Remove from heat. Add cream cheese. Mix well using a wire whisk until well blended. Pour hot mixture evenly over bananas. Evenly sprinkle graham cracker crumbs over top. Refrigerate for at least 1 hour. Cut into 8 servings. When serving, top each piece with 1 tablespoon Cool Whip Lite.

HINTS: 1. To prevent banana from turning brown, mix with
            1 teaspoon lemon juice or sprinkle with Fruit Fresh.
         2. A self-seal sandwich bag works great for crushing
            graham crackers.

Each serving equals:

HE: ½ Bread • ½ Vegetable • ½ Protein • ¼ Fruit •
1 Slider • 3 Optional Calories

182 Calories • 6 gm Fat • 6 gm Protein •
26 gm Carbohydrate • 402 mg Sodium •
28 mg Calcium • 1 gm Fiber

DIABETIC: 1 Starch/Carbohydrate • 1 Fat • ½ Fruit •
½ Meat

Layered Coconut Banana Cream Pie

Just like one of my most popular desserts, the Triple Layer Party Pie (*Healthy Exchanges Cookbook*), this tropical treasure features three scrumptious layers that add up to one sensational pie! Close your eyes, take a bite, and you're almost in Hawaii. . . .

🌀 Serves 8

> 1 (8-ounce) package Philadelphia fat-free cream cheese
> 1 cup Cool Whip Free☆
> 1 teaspoon coconut extract☆
> 1 (4-serving) package JELL-O sugar-free orange gelatin☆
> 1 (6-ounce) Keebler graham cracker piecrust
> 1 (4-serving) package JELL-O sugar-free instant banana cream pudding mix
> ⅔ cup Carnation Nonfat Dry Milk Powder
> 1¼ cups water
> 1⅓ cups (2 small) diced bananas
> 2 tablespoons flaked coconut

In a large bowl, stir cream cheese with a spoon until soft. Add ¼ cup Cool Whip Free, ½ teaspoon coconut extract, and 1 tablespoon dry gelatin. Mix well to combine. Spread mixture evenly into piecrust. In a medium bowl, combine dry pudding mix, dry milk powder, and water. Mix well using a wire whisk. Fold in bananas. Spread banana mixture evenly over cream cheese mixture. In a small bowl, combine remaining ¾ cup Cool Whip Free, remaining ½ teaspoon coconut extract, and remaining dry gelatin. Spread mixture evenly over banana mixture. Sprinkle coconut evenly over top. Refrigerate for at least 1 hour. Cut into 8 servings.

HINT: To prevent bananas from turning brown, mix with 1 teaspoon lemon juice or sprinkle with Fruit Fresh.

Each serving equals:

HE: ½ Bread • ½ Protein • ½ Fruit • 1 Slider •
7 Optional Calories

214 Calories • 6 gm Fat • 8 gm Protein •
32 gm Carbohydrate • 541 mg Sodium •
71 mg Calcium • 1 gm Fiber

DIABETIC: 1½ Starch • 1 Fat • ½ Fruit
or 2 Starch/Carbohydrate • 1 Fat

John's Apple Crumb Pie

I created this tasty concoction for my son-in-law, John, who loves apple pie. I figured it wouldn't take Becky long to whip this one up, even if cooking is not one of her favorite hobbies. When it comes to special occasions like birthdays, she gladly dons her apron and aims to please! ◐ Serves 8

> 1 (4-serving) package JELL-O sugar-free vanilla cook-and-serve pudding mix
>
> 1 cup unsweetened apple juice
>
> ¼ cup water
>
> 1 teaspoon apple pie spice
>
> 3 cups (6 small) cored, unpeeled, and diced cooking apples
>
> 1 (6-ounce) Keebler graham cracker piecrust
>
> 6 tablespoons purchased graham cracker crumbs or 6 (2½-inch) graham cracker squares made into crumbs
>
> 1 tablespoon Brown Sugar Twin
>
> 2 tablespoons (½ ounce) chopped pecans

Preheat oven to 375 degrees. In a large saucepan, combine dry pudding mix, apple juice, water, and apple pie spice. Stir in apples. Cook over medium heat until apples soften and mixture starts to boil, stirring often. Spoon hot apple mixture into piecrust. In a medium bowl, combine graham cracker crumbs, Brown Sugar Twin, and pecans. Sprinkle crumb mixture evenly over top. Bake for 18 to 22 minutes. Place pie plate on a wire rack and allow to cool for at least 30 minutes. Cut into 8 servings.

HINTS: 1. A self-seal sandwich bag works great for crushing graham crackers.

2. Good served warm or cold. Also tasty with either Cool Whip Lite or sugar- and fat-free vanilla ice cream, but don't forget to count the few additional calories.

Each serving equals:

HE: 1 Fruit • ¾ Bread • ¼ Fat • ¾ Slider •
1 Optional Calorie

---

195 Calories • 7 gm Fat • 2 gm Protein •
31 gm Carbohydrate • 227 mg Sodium •
7 mg Calcium • 2 gm Fiber

DIABETIC: 1 Fruit • 1 Starch • 1 Fat
or 2 Starch/Carbohydrate • 1 Fat

Peach Blueberry Pie

There's something magical about fresh fruit pies, maybe because the season for certain fruits (like peaches and blueberries, for instance) just isn't all that long. Choose the ripest, most perfect fruit you can find, invite the people you love most to join you, and celebrate the flavors of summer in every bite!   ☻   Serves 8

> 1 (8-ounce) package Philadelphia fat-free cream cheese
> Sugar substitute to equal 2 tablespoons sugar
> 1 teaspoon vanilla extract
> 1½ cups fresh blueberries
> 1 (6-ounce) Keebler shortbread piecrust
> Water☆
> 2 cups (4 medium) peeled and sliced fresh peaches
> 1 (4-serving) package JELL-O sugar-free vanilla cook-and-serve
>   pudding mix
> ½ cup Cool Whip Lite

In a medium bowl, stir cream cheese with a spoon until soft. Add sugar substitute and vanilla extract. Mix well to combine. Gently fold in blueberries. Spread mixture evenly into piecrust. Place ¼ cup water and peaches in a blender container. Cover and process on HIGH until mixture is smooth. Add enough water to mixture to make 1½ cups liquid. Mix well to combine. In a medium saucepan, combine dry pudding mix and blended peach mixture. Cook over medium heat until mixture thickens and starts to boil, stirring often. Remove from heat. Place saucepan on a wire rack and allow to cool for 10 minutes. Spoon pudding mixture evenly over cream cheese mixture. Refrigerate for at least 2 hours. Cut into 8 servings. When serving, top each piece with 1 tablespoon Cool Whip Lite.

Each serving equals:

HE: ¾ Fruit • ½ Bread • ½ Protein • ¾ Slider •
10 Optional Calories

---

182 Calories • 6 gm Fat • 5 gm Protein •
27 gm Carbohydrate • 364 mg Sodium •
4 mg Calcium • 2 gm Fiber

DIABETIC: 1 Fruit • 1 Starch • 1 Fat • ½ Meat

Orange Pecan Pie

I'm nuts about pecans—everyone knows it—and so I'm fond of finding ways to stir them into everything from salads to desserts. The ingredients in this scrumptious pie might seem an unusual partnership, but take a chance on this one—you won't be sorry!

● Serves 8

> 1 (4-serving) package JELL-O sugar-free vanilla cook-and-serve pudding mix
> 1 (4-serving) package JELL-O sugar-free orange gelatin
> 1½ cups water
> 1 cup (one 11-ounce can) mandarin oranges, rinsed and drained
> 6 tablespoons (1½ ounces) chopped pecans
> 1 (6-ounce) Keebler graham cracker piecrust
> 2 tablespoons purchased graham cracker crumbs or two (2½-inch) graham cracker squares made into crumbs

In a large saucepan, combine dry pudding mix, dry gelatin, and water. Cook over medium heat until mixture thickens and starts to boil, stirring constantly. Remove from heat. Gently stir in mandarin oranges and pecans. Spoon hot mixture into piecrust. Refrigerate for at least 2 hours. Evenly sprinkle graham cracker crumbs over top. Cut into 8 servings.

HINT: A self-seal sandwich bag works great for crushing graham crackers.

Each serving equals:

HE: ¾ Fat • ½ Bread • ¼ Fruit • ¾ Slider • 12 Optional Calories

177 Calories • 9 gm Fat • 2 gm Protein • 22 gm Carbohydrate • 233 mg Sodium • 6 mg Calcium • 1 gm Fiber

DIABETIC: 1½ Starch/Carbohydrate • 1 Fat

Frosty Pumpkin Ice Cream Pie

When Shirley, my friend and faithful typist since the beginning of Healthy Exchanges, asked me to "skinny up" her favorite holiday pie, I said I'd do my best, and here it is: nutty and sweet, cool and creamy, and proof that great desserts can be healthy too!

○ Serves 8

> 2 cups Wells' Blue Bunny sugar- and fat-free vanilla ice cream or
>   any sugar- and fat-free ice cream
> 2 cups (one 16-ounce can) pumpkin
> ¼ cup Sugar Twin or Sprinkle Sweet
> ¼ cup Brown Sugar Twin
> 1½ teaspoons pumpkin pie spice
> 1 (6-ounce) Keebler graham cracker piecrust
> ½ cup Cool Whip Lite
> 2 tablespoons (½ ounce) chopped pecans

In a large bowl, stir ice cream to soften. Add pumpkin, Sugar Twin, Brown Sugar Twin, and pumpkin pie spice. Mix well using a wire whisk. Evenly spread mixture into piecrust. Cover and freeze. Remove from freezer 10 to 15 minutes before serving. Cut into 8 servings. When serving, top each piece with 1 tablespoon Cool Whip Lite and ¾ teaspoon pecans.

Each serving equals:

HE: ½ Bread • ¼ Vegetable • ¼ Fat • 1 Slider •
10 Optional Calories

---

182 Calories • 6 gm Fat • 4 gm Protein •
28 gm Carbohydrate • 163 mg Sodium •
77 mg Calcium • 2 gm Fiber

DIABETIC: 1½ Starch/Carbohydrate • 1 Fat

Black Bottom Pumpkin Cream Pie

Here's another frightfully festive Halloween treat that's definitely no trick! If you're looking for a yummy dessert matched perfectly to your orange-and-black holiday decorations, look no further than this gleefully ghostly pie. ☻ Serves 8

> 1 (8-ounce) package Philadelphia fat-free cream cheese☆
> 1 (4-serving) package JELL-O sugar-free instant chocolate pudding mix
> 1⅓ cups Carnation Nonfat Dry Milk Powder☆
> 1¼ cups water☆
> 1 (6-ounce) Keebler chocolate piecrust
> 1 (4-serving) package JELL-O sugar-free instant vanilla pudding mix
> 2 cups (one 16-ounce can) pumpkin
> 1 teaspoon pumpkin pie spice
> ¾ cup Cool Whip Lite☆

Place 4 ounces (half of package) of cream cheese in a large bowl and stir with a spoon until soft. Add dry chocolate pudding mix, ⅔ cup dry milk powder, and 1 cup water. Mix well using a wire whisk. Evenly spread mixture into piecrust. In another large bowl, stir remaining 4 ounces cream cheese until soft. Add dry vanilla pudding mix, remaining ⅔ cup dry milk powder, remaining ¼ cup water, and pumpkin. Mix well using a wire whisk. Blend in pumpkin pie spice and ¼ cup Cool Whip Lite. Spread pumpkin mixture evenly over chocolate layer. Refrigerate for at least 1 hour. Cut into 8 servings. When serving, top each piece with 1 tablespoon Cool Whip Lite.

Each serving equals:

HE: ½ Bread • ½ Protein • ½ Skim Milk •
¼ Vegetable • 1 Slider • 13 Optional Calories

---

222 Calories • 6 gm Fat • 10 gm Protein •
32 gm Carbohydrate • 653 mg Sodium •
155 mg Calcium • 3 gm Fiber

DIABETIC: 1½ Starch • 1 Fat • ½ Meat • ½ Skim Milk
or 2 Starch/Carbohydrate • 1 Fat • ½ Meat

Lemon Supreme Cheesecake Pie

Can anything as delectable as my healthy cheesecakes truly be good for you? Fear not, they're low in fat and rich in flavors so tasty you'll be sure you've gone to heaven after just one bite! This lemon one is just right for a bridal shower or garden party, maybe because it tastes light and rich all at once! ☻ Serves 8

> 2 (8-ounce) packages Philadelphia fat-free cream cheese
> 1 (4-serving) package JELL-O sugar-free instant vanilla pudding mix
> ⅔ cup Carnation Nonfat Dry Milk Powder
> 2 (4-serving) packages JELL-O sugar-free lemon gelatin☆
> 2 cups Diet Mountain Dew☆
> 1 (6-ounce) Keebler shortbread piecrust
> 1 (4-serving) package JELL-O sugar-free vanilla cook-and-serve pudding mix
> 1 cup Cool Whip Lite☆

In a large bowl, stir cream cheese with a spoon until soft. Add dry instant pudding mix, dry milk powder, 1 package dry gelatin, and 1 cup Diet Mountain Dew. Mix well using a wire whisk. Spread mixture evenly into piecrust. Refrigerate. Meanwhile, in a medium saucepan, combine dry cook-and-serve pudding mix, remaining package dry gelatin, and remaining 1 cup Diet Mountain Dew. Cook over medium heat until mixture thickens and starts to boil, stirring constantly. Remove from heat. Place pan on a wire rack and allow to cool for 30 minutes. Blend in ½ cup Cool Whip Lite. Spread pudding mixture evenly over cheesecake mixture. Refrigerate for at least 1 hour. Cut into 8 servings. When serving, top each piece with 1 tablespoon Cool Whip Lite.

Each serving equals:

HE: 1 Protein • ½ Bread • ¼ Skim Milk • 1 Slider • 18 Optional Calories

205 Calories • 5 gm Fat • 12 gm Protein • 28 gm Carbohydrate • 681 mg Sodium • 69 mg Calcium • 1 gm Fiber

DIABETIC: 2 Starch/Carbohydrate • 1 Meat • 1 Fat

Raspberry-Almond Cheesecake

It's simple, it's elegant, and it's special enough to serve at a wedding or anniversary party, anytime when you want to show people just how much you care for them. Isn't it great to know you can prepare a luxurious dessert like this one only an hour or so before a special event?   ☺   Serves 8

> 2 (8-ounce) packages Philadelphia fat-free cream cheese
> 1 (4-serving) package JELL-O sugar-free instant vanilla pudding
>   mix
> ²⁄₃ cup Carnation Nonfat Dry Milk Powder
> 1 cup Diet Mountain Dew
> ³⁄₄ cup Cool Whip Free☆
> 1 teaspoon almond extract☆
> 1 (6-ounce) Keebler shortbread piecrust
> ½ cup raspberry spreadable fruit
> 2 tablespoons (½ ounce) slivered almonds

In a large bowl, stir cream cheese with a spoon until soft. Add dry pudding mix, dry milk powder, and Diet Mountain Dew. Mix well using a wire whisk. Blend in ¼ cup Cool Whip Free and ½ teaspoon almond extract. Spread mixture evenly into piecrust. In a small bowl, stir spreadable fruit until soft. Add remaining ½ cup Cool Whip Free and remaining ½ teaspoon almond extract. Mix gently to combine. Spread topping mixture evenly over filling mixture. Evenly sprinkle almonds over top. Refrigerate for at least 1 hour. Cut into 8 servings.

Each serving equals:

HE: 1 Protein • 1 Fruit • ½ Bread • ¼ Skim Milk •
1 Slider • 9 Optional Calories

238 Calories • 6 gm Fat • 11 gm Protein •
35 gm Carbohydrate • 678 mg Sodium •
75 mg Calcium • 1 gm Fiber

DIABETIC: 1 Starch • 1 Meat • 1 Fruit • 1 Fat

Taffy Apple Cheesecake

There's nothing like the flavors of sweet childhood memories grown ever sweeter as time has passed. This dessert offers you the chance to relive those happy days in every single scrumptious bite, from the caramel and nuts to the mouth-pleasing crunch of the apples!

○ Serves 8

> 2 (8-ounce) packages Philadelphia fat-free cream cheese
> 1 (4-serving) package JELL-O sugar-free instant vanilla pudding mix
> ⅔ cup Carnation Nonfat Dry Milk Powder
> 1 cup unsweetened apple juice
> ¼ cup Cool Whip Free
> 2 tablespoons caramel syrup
> 1 cup (2 small) cored, unpeeled, and finely diced Red Delicious apples
> ¼ cup (1 ounce) chopped dry-roasted peanuts☆
> 1 (6-ounce) Keebler graham cracker piecrust

In a large bowl, stir cream cheese with a spoon until soft. Add dry pudding mix, dry milk powder, and apple juice. Mix well using a wire whisk. Blend in Cool Whip Free and caramel syrup. Gently stir in apples and 2 tablespoons peanuts. Spread mixture into piecrust. Evenly sprinkle remaining 2 tablespoons peanuts over top. Refrigerate for at least 1 hour. Cut into 8 servings.

Each serving equals:

HE: 1 Protein • ½ Bread • ½ Fruit • ¼ Skim Milk • ¼ Fat • 1 Slider • 3 Optional Calories

---

235 Calories • 7 gm Fat • 12 gm Protein • 31 gm Carbohydrate • 690 mg Sodium • 78 mg Calcium • 1 gm Fiber

---

DIABETIC: 1½ Starch • 1 Meat • 1 Fat • ½ Fruit *or* 2 Starch/Carbohydrate • 1 Meat • 1 Fat

Rum Raisin Cheesecake

I don't know who first thought of blending the wild taste of the Caribbean with the super-sweet flavor of raisins, but I figure they ought to get a medal of some kind—or at least, a cheesecake! If rum raisin is your flavor of choice, now you've got another scrumptious way to enjoy it.   ○   Serves 8

> 2 (8-ounce) packages Philadelphia fat-free cream cheese
> 1 (4-serving) package JELL-O sugar-free instant vanilla pudding mix
> 2/3 cup Carnation Nonfat Dry Milk Powder
> 1 cup water
> 1 cup Cool Whip Free☆
> 1½ teaspoons rum extract☆
> ¼ cup (1 ounce) chopped walnuts☆
> ½ cup raisins
> 1 (6-ounce) Keebler shortbread piecrust

In a large bowl, stir cream cheese with a spoon until soft. Add dry pudding mix, dry milk powder, and water. Mix well to combine. Blend in ¼ cup Cool Whip Free and 1 teaspoon rum extract. Add 2 tablespoons walnuts and raisins. Mix gently to combine. Spread mixture evenly into piecrust. Refrigerate while preparing topping. In a small bowl, combine remaining ¾ cup Cool Whip Free and remaining ½ teaspoon rum extract. Spread topping mixture evenly over set filling. Evenly sprinkle remaining walnuts over top. Refrigerate for at least 1 hour. Cut into 8 servings.

HINT: To plump up raisins without "cooking," place in a glass measuring cup and microwave on HIGH for 20 seconds.

Each serving equals:

HE: 1 Protein • ½ Bread • ½ Fruit • ¼ Fat •
¼ Skim Milk • 1 Slider • 10 Optional Calories

240 Calories • 8 gm Fat • 12 gm Protein •
30 gm Carbohydrate • 672 mg Sodium •
77 mg Calcium • 1 gm Fiber

DIABETIC: 2 Starch/Carbohydrate • 1 Meat • 1 Fat

Orange Chocolate Crumb Cheesecake

A friend once told me about a retired ice cream flavor that blended oranges and chocolate, and my mind started creating this wonderful cheesecake on the spot! Sweet and tangy, fruity and crunchy, it provides an abundance of taste sensations you'll never forget.

Serves 8

> 2 (8-ounce) packages Philadelphia fat-free cream cheese
> 1 (4-serving) package JELL-O sugar-free instant vanilla pudding mix
> 2/3 cup Carnation Nonfat Dry Milk Powder
> 1 cup unsweetened orange juice
> 1/2 cup Cool Whip Free
> 1 cup (one 11-ounce can) mandarin oranges, rinsed and drained
> 6 (2 1/2-inch) chocolate graham crackers made into crumbs☆
> 1 (6-ounce) Keebler chocolate piecrust

In a large bowl, stir cream cheese with a spoon until soft. Add dry pudding mix, dry milk powder, and orange juice. Mix well using a wire whisk. Blend in Cool Whip Free and mandarin oranges. Gently fold in 1/4 cup graham cracker crumbs. Spread mixture into piecrust. Evenly sprinkle remaining 2 tablespoons graham cracker crumbs over top. Refrigerate for at least 1 hour. Cut into 8 servings.

HINT: A self-seal sandwich bag works great for crushing graham crackers.

Each serving equals:

HE: 1 Protein • ¾ Bread • ½ Fruit • ¼ Skim Milk • ¾ Slider • 13 Optional Calories

---

234 Calories • 6 gm Fat • 12 gm Protein • 33 gm Carbohydrate • 584 mg Sodium • 67 mg Calcium • 1 gm Fiber

---

DIABETIC: 1½ Starch • 1 Meat • ½ Fruit • 1 Fat *or* 2 Starch/Carbohydrate • 1 Meat • 1 Fat

Black Forest Cheesecake

Would you believe that instead of a classic wedding cake, one young bride I knew opted to fly in a dozen chocolate-cherry cheesecakes from a famous New York bakery? I'm not all that surprised. The combination of flavors known as "Black Forest" are simply irresistible! ☾ Serves 8

> 1 (4-serving) package JELL-O sugar-free cherry gelatin
> 1 (4-serving) package JELL-O sugar-free vanilla cook-and-serve
>   pudding mix
> 1½ cups water☆
> 2 cups (one 16-ounce can) tart red cherries, packed in water,
>   undrained
> 1 teaspoon almond extract
> 2 (8-ounce) packages Philadelphia fat-free cream cheese
> 1 (4-serving) package JELL-O sugar-free instant chocolate
>   pudding mix
> ⅔ cup Carnation Nonfat Dry Milk Powder
> 1 (6-ounce) Keebler chocolate piecrust
> ½ cup Cool Whip Lite
> 1 tablespoon + 1 teaspoon (⅓ ounce) mini chocolate chips

In a medium saucepan, combine dry gelatin and dry cook-and-serve pudding mix. Add ½ cup water and undrained cherries. Mix gently to combine. Cook over medium heat until mixture thickens and starts to boil, stirring constantly, being careful not to crush cherries. Remove from heat. Stir in almond extract. Place saucepan on a wire rack and allow to cool for 30 minutes. Meanwhile, in a large bowl, stir cream cheese with a spoon until soft. Add dry instant pudding mix, dry milk powder, and remaining 1 cup water. Mix well using a wire whisk. Spread pudding mixture into piecrust. Refrigerate until cherry mixture has cooled. Evenly spoon cooled cherry mixture over chocolate layer. Drop Cool Whip Lite by tablespoonful to form 8 mounds. Evenly sprinkle about

½ teaspoon chocolate chips over top of each mound. Refrigerate for at least 1 hour. Cut into 8 servings.

Each serving equals:

HE: 1 Protein • ½ Bread • ½ Fruit • 1 Slider • 17 Optional Calories

234 Calories • 6 gm Fat • 13 gm Protein • 33 gm Carbohydrate • 725 mg Sodium • 77 mg Calcium • 1 gm Fiber

DIABETIC: 1½ Starch • 1 Meat • 1 Fat • ½ Fruit

Mocha Mint Cake Dessert

This blend of flavors might strike you as unusual, but you'll be pleasantly surprised at how well they fit together! The coffee seems to make the chocolate even more intense than it is on its own.

♥ Serves 12

  1½ cups all-purpose flour
  ¼ cup unsweetened cocoa
  ½ cup Sugar Twin or Sprinkle Sweet
  1 cup Carnation Nonfat Dry Milk Powder☆
  1 teaspoon baking powder
  1 teaspoon baking soda
  ⅔ cup Kraft fat-free mayonnaise
  2 cups cold coffee☆
  2 teaspoons mint extract☆
  1 (4-serving) package JELL-O sugar-free instant chocolate fudge
     pudding mix
  1½ cups Cool Whip Free
  5 to 6 drops green food coloring
  2 tablespoons (½ ounce) mini chocolate chips

Preheat oven to 350 degrees. Spray a 9-by-9-inch cake pan with butter-flavored cooking spray. In a large bowl, combine flour, cocoa, Sugar Twin, ⅓ cup dry milk powder, baking powder, and baking soda. Add mayonnaise, 1 cup cold coffee, and 1 teaspoon mint extract. Mix well to combine. Pour batter into prepared cake pan. Bake for 18 to 22 minutes or until a toothpick inserted in center comes out clean. Gently punch holes in top of cake with tines of a fork. Place cake pan on a wire rack and allow to cool for 10 minutes. In a medium bowl, combine dry pudding mix, remaining ⅔ cup dry milk powder, and remaining 1 cup cold coffee. Mix well using a wire whisk. Spread pudding mixture evenly over partially cooled cake. Continue cooling for 15 minutes. In a small bowl, combine Cool Whip Free, remaining 1 teaspoon mint extract, and green food coloring. Spread topping mixture evenly over chocolate pudding layer. Sprinkle chocolate chips evenly over top. Cut into 12 servings. Refrigerate leftovers.

Each serving equals:

HE: ⅔ Bread • ¼ Skim Milk • ½ Slider •
17 Optional Calories

129 Calories • 1 gm Fat • 4 gm Protein •
26 gm Carbohydrate • 403 mg Sodium •
98 mg Calcium • 1 gm Fiber

DIABETIC: 1½ Starch/Carbohydrate *or*
1 Starch/Carbohydrate • ½ Skim Milk

Mocha Roll

This chocolate-coffee pudding cake is wonderfully rich and moist, a terrific choice to follow a spicy Mexican meal. If you've never made a jelly-roll-style cake before, don't worry—just take your time gently rolling it up. ☻ Serves 8

> *4 eggs or equivalent in egg substitute*
>
> *1 teaspoon vanilla extract*
>
> *½ cup Sugar Twin or Sprinkle Sweet*
>
> *¾ cup Aunt Jemima Reduced Fat Pancake Mix*
>
> *1 (4-serving) package JELL-O sugar-free instant chocolate fudge pudding mix*
>
> *⅔ cup Carnation Nonfat Dry Milk Powder*
>
> *2 teaspoons instant coffee crystals*
>
> *1¼ cups water*
>
> *⅓ cup Cool Whip Free*
>
> *1 tablespoon + 1 teaspoon powdered sugar (optional)*

Preheat oven to 400 degrees. Line a 15½-by-10½-by-1-inch pan with waxed paper and spray paper with butter-flavored cooking spray. In a blender container, combine eggs and vanilla extract. Cover and process on BLEND until frothy. Add Sugar Twin. Continue processing on BLEND until smooth. Add pancake mix. Process on BLEND until combined. Pour mixture into prepared pan. Bake for 6 to 8 minutes. Loosen sides with a knife. Place a clean cloth over top, turn pan over and gently shake cake loose from pan. Carefully peel waxed paper from cake. Starting at narrow end, roll cake with towel inside. Cool for 30 minutes. In a medium bowl, combine dry pudding mix, dry milk powder, and coffee crystals. Add water. Mix well using a wire whisk. Blend in Cool Whip Free. Gently unroll cooled cake. Remove towel. Spread pudding mixture evenly over cake. Re-roll. Place on a serving plate, seam side down, and refrigerate for at least 30 minutes. Cut into 8 pieces. When serving, sprinkle top of each piece with ½ teaspoon powdered sugar, if desired.

Each serving equals:

HE: ½ Bread • ½ Protein (limited) • ¼ Skim Milk •
¼ Slider • 8 Optional Calories

131 Calories • 3 gm Fat • 8 gm Protein •
18 gm Carbohydrate • 374 mg Sodium •
150 mg Calcium • 2 gm Fiber

DIABETIC: 1 Starch/Carbohydrate • ½ Meat

Pineapple Spice Cake

Spice cake is one of Cliff's favorite desserts, so over the years, I've come up with many different combinations of flavors to please him. This pineapple version is one of the sweetest and creamiest I've tried. My grandbaby Josh, who loves pineapple so much, also gobbled it down with a big smile! ☻ Serves 8

1½ cups all-purpose flour

½ cup Sugar Twin or Sprinkle Sweet

1 teaspoon baking powder

1 teaspoon baking soda

1½ teaspoons apple pie spice

½ cup raisins

2 cups (two 8-ounce cans) crushed pineapple, packed in fruit juice, undrained☆

1 cup Diet Mountain Dew☆

2 teaspoons coconut extract☆

½ cup Yoplait plain fat-free yogurt

⅓ cup Kraft fat-free mayonnaise

1 (4-serving) package JELL-O sugar-free instant vanilla pudding mix

⅔ cup Carnation Nonfat Dry Milk Powder

1 cup Cool Whip Free

2 tablespoons flaked coconut

Preheat oven to 350 degrees. Spray a 9-by-9-inch cake pan with butter-flavored cooking spray. In a large bowl, combine flour, Sugar Twin, baking powder, baking soda, and apple pie spice. Stir in raisins. In a medium bowl, combine 1 cup undrained pineapple, ½ cup Diet Mountain Dew, 1 teaspoon coconut extract, yogurt, and mayonnaise. Mix well until blended. Add pineapple mixture to flour mixture. Mix gently just until combined. Spread batter into prepared cake pan. Bake for 25 to 30 minutes or until a toothpick inserted in center comes out clean. Place cake pan on a wire rack and allow to cool completely. In a medium bowl, combine dry pudding mix, dry milk powder, remaining 1 cup undrained pineapple, and remaining ½ cup Diet Mountain Dew. Mix well using a wire whisk. Blend in remaining 1 teaspoon coconut extract and Cool Whip Free. Spread mixture evenly over cooled cake. Evenly sprinkle coconut over top. Cut into 8 servings. Refrigerate leftovers.

Each serving equals:

HE: 1 Bread • 1 Fruit • ⅓ Skim Milk • ½ Slider •
9 Optional Calories

221 Calories • 1 gm Fat • 6 gm Protein •
47 gm Carbohydrate • 507 mg Sodium •
148 mg Calcium • 2 gm Fiber

DIABETIC: 2 Starch/Carbohydrate • 1 Fruit

This and That

Florida Orange Dressing

This delicious fruity blend may surprise your family the first time they taste it, but it works beautifully on a salad of tender lettuce like Boston or Bibb. You may want to add a few mandarin oranges as a garnish.　●　Serves 6 (3 tablespoons)

½ cup unsweetened orange juice
3 tablespoons sugar-free orange marmalade
¾ cup Kraft fat-free mayonnaise

In a small bowl, combine orange juice and orange marmalade. Add mayonnaise. Mix well to combine. Cover and refrigerate for at least 30 minutes.

Each serving equals:

HE: ½ Fruit • ¼ Slider

40 Calories • 0 gm Fat • 0 gm Protein •
10 gm Carbohydrate • 215 mg Sodium •
5 mg Calcium • 0 gm Fiber

DIABETIC: ½ Fruit *or* ½ Starch/Carbohydrate

Sam's Creamy Mustard Garlic Dressing

I created this for one of the most loyal listeners our radio show has ever had. When she called up to ask for a creamy garlic dressing, I was happy to oblige. Just remember not to serve it on those nights when romance is also on the menu!

○ Serves 8 (2 tablespoons)

> ¾ cup Kraft fat-free mayonnaise
> 1 tablespoon Dijon mustard
> ¼ cup skim milk
> Sugar substitute to equal 2 teaspoons sugar
> 1 tablespoon white vinegar
> 1 teaspoon dried minced garlic
> 1 teaspoon dried parsley flakes

In a small bowl, combine mayonnaise, mustard, skim milk, sugar substitute, and vinegar. Add garlic and parsley flakes. Mix well to combine. Cover and refrigerate. Gently stir again just before serving.

Each serving equals:

HE: ¼ Slider

20 Calories • 0 gm Fat • 0 gm Protein •
5 gm Carbohydrate • 247 mg Sodium •
13 mg Calcium • 0 gm Fiber

DIABETIC: Free food

Ranchero Sauce

Here's a lively sauce just right to pour over omelets, hamburgers, and even grilled chicken. If you like to barbecue, try brushing it on whatever you're grilling, even vegetables, and see how great they taste! ○ Serves 4 (⅓ cup)

½ cup sliced onion
¼ cup chopped green bell pepper
1 (10¾-ounce) can Healthy Request Tomato Soup
1 teaspoon chili seasoning
½ cup (one 2.5-ounce jar) sliced mushrooms, undrained
¼ cup (one 2-ounce jar) chopped pimiento, undrained

In a large skillet sprayed with olive oil–flavored cooking spray, sauté onion and green pepper for 5 minutes or until tender. Stir in tomato soup and chili seasoning. Add mushrooms and pimiento. Mix well to combine. Lower heat and simmer for 5 minutes, stirring occasionally.

Each serving equals:

HE: ¾ Vegetable • ½ Slider • 5 Optional Calories

---

65 Calories • 1 gm Fat • 2 gm Protein •
12 gm Carbohydrate • 315 mg Sodium •
15 mg Calcium • 2 gm Fiber

DIABETIC: 1 Vegetable • ½ Starch

Festive Spinach Dip

Everyone needs perfect party foods, and this dip found lots of fans when I tested it recently. Try it with carrot or celery sticks, or perhaps some of the healthy baked chips you find in just about every market these days.   ☻   Serves 8 (⅓ cup)

> 1 (8-ounce) package Philadelphia fat-free cream cheese
> ½ cup Land O Lakes no-fat sour cream
> ½ cup Kraft Fat Free Ranch Dressing
> 1 teaspoon dried onion flakes
> ¼ cup (one 2-ounce jar) chopped pimiento
> 1 (10-ounce) package frozen chopped spinach, thawed and well
>   drained
> 1 (8-ounce) can water chestnuts, drained and chopped

In a medium bowl, stir cream cheese with a spoon until soft. Stir in sour cream, Ranch dressing, onion flakes, and pimiento. Add spinach and water chestnuts. Mix well to combine. Cover and refrigerate for at least 30 minutes. Gently stir again just before serving.

Each serving equals:

HE: ½ Protein • ½ Vegetable • ¼ Bread • ¼ Slider

---

80 Calories • 0 gm Fat • 6 gm Protein •
14 gm Carbohydrate • 379 mg Sodium •
57 mg Calcium • 2 gm Fiber

DIABETIC: 1 Starch/Carbohydrate • ½ Meat

Mexican Eggs

Instead of pouring hot sauce over your eggs for an eye-opener, give this dish a try! By stirring the salsa right in, you'll get a real fiesta of flavors to help you start the day!   ☻   Serves 4

> 1 cup chunky salsa (mild, medium, or hot)
> ¼ cup Heinz Light Harvest Ketchup or any reduced-sodium ketchup
> ¼ cup water
> 4 eggs or equivalent in egg substitute
> 2 tablespoons chopped fresh parsley or 2 teaspoons dried parsley flakes

In a large skillet, combine salsa, ketchup, and water. Cook over medium heat until mixture starts to boil. Break eggs into skillet. Lower heat, cover, and simmer until eggs are cooked to desired doneness, basting once or twice while simmering. Just before serving, sprinkle parsley over top. Divide into 4 servings.

Each serving equals:

HE: 1 Protein (limited) • ½ Vegetable • ¼ Slider • 10 Optional Calories

89 Calories • 5 gm Fat • 6 gm Protein • 5 gm Carbohydrate • 399 mg Sodium • 108 mg Calcium • 0 gm Fiber

DIABETIC: 1 Meat • 1 Vegetable

Border Scramble

Here's a great hearty entree to serve at your next weekend brunch! Tasty and tangy, chock-full of favorite flavors, and as spicy as you want it to be, this is wonderful for lunch or supper as well. And it looks as if you had to get up at the crack of dawn to fix it, but its ease of preparation can be our little secret.   ☺   Serves 4

8 ounces ground 90% lean turkey or beef
½ teaspoon poultry seasoning
¼ teaspoon ground sage
¼ teaspoon garlic powder
1½ cups (8 ounces) diced cooked potatoes
½ cup chopped onion
1 cup chopped fresh tomatoes

½ cup chopped green bell pepper
1 cup chunky salsa (mild, medium, or hot)
4 (6-inch) flour tortillas
⅓ cup (1½ ounces) shredded Kraft reduced-fat Cheddar cheese
¼ cup Land O Lakes no-fat sour cream

In a large skillet sprayed with butter-flavored cooking spray, brown meat with poultry seasoning, sage, and garlic powder. Add potatoes, onion, tomatoes, green pepper, and salsa. Lower heat, cover, and simmer for 10 minutes. For each serving, place 1 tortilla on a serving plate, spoon about ¾ cup meat mixture over top and garnish with full 1 tablespoon Cheddar cheese and 1 tablespoon sour cream. Serve at once.

HINT: I didn't peel either the potatoes or tomatoes, but do so if you wish.

Each serving equals:

HE: 2 Protein • 1½ Bread • 1½ Vegetable • 15 Optional Calories

288 Calories • 8 gm Fat • 18 gm Protein • 36 gm Carbohydrate • 399 mg Sodium • 186 mg Calcium • 3 gm Fiber

DIABETIC: 2 Meat • 2 Starch • 1 Vegetable

Biscuit Brunch Boats

Kids really love these biscuit cups piled high with creamy eggs and cheese, but I doubt anyone of any age would say no when you bring these "boats" to the table. Happy sailing!   ❤   Serves 5

1 (7.5-ounce) can Pillsbury refrigerated buttermilk biscuits
5 eggs or equivalent in egg substitute
½ cup skim milk☆
½ teaspoon lemon pepper
2 tablespoons Hormel Bacon Bits
1 (10¾-ounce) can Healthy Request Cream of Mushroom Soup
⅔ cup (2¼ ounces) shredded Kraft reduced-fat Cheddar cheese
1 teaspoon dried parsley flakes

Preheat oven to 375 degrees. Spray 10 wells of a 12-hole muffin pan with butter-flavored cooking spray. Separate biscuits and pat each into a prepared muffin well. In a medium bowl, combine eggs, 2 tablespoons skim milk, lemon pepper, and bacon bits. Evenly spoon mixture into biscuit "boats." Bake for 15 minutes or until eggs are set. Meanwhile, in a medium saucepan, combine mushroom soup, remaining 6 tablespoons skim milk, Cheddar cheese, and parsley flakes. Cook over medium-low heat until cheese melts and "boats" are done. For each serving, place 2 "boats" on a plate and spoon about ⅓ cup cheese sauce over top.

HINT: Fill unused muffin wells with water. It protects the muffin tin and ensures even baking.

Each serving equals:

HE: 1⅔ Protein (1 limited) • 1½ Bread • ½ Slider •
14 Optional Calories

266 Calories • 10 gm Fat • 16 gm Protein •
28 gm Carbohydrate • 913 mg Sodium •
180 mg Calcium • 2 gm Fiber

DIABETIC: 2 Starch • 1½ Meat

Mini Focaccia Biscuits

If you haven't tried the crusty Italian bread brushed with flavored oil and herbs, you've got something very tasty coming! These are almost like mini-pizzas without the tomato sauce.

◐ Serves 6

> 1 (7.5-ounce) can Pillsbury refrigerated biscuits
> 1/4 cup (3/4 ounce) grated Kraft fat-free Parmesan cheese
> 1 1/2 teaspoons dried basil
> 1 teaspoon dried parsley flakes
> 1/2 teaspoon dried minced garlic
> 1/3 cup Kraft Fat Free Italian Dressing
> 3/4 cup finely chopped fresh tomatoes
> 1/3 cup (1 1/2 ounces) shredded Kraft reduced-fat mozzarella cheese

Preheat oven to 400 degrees. Spray a deep-dish 10-inch pie plate with olive oil–flavored cooking spray. Separate biscuits and cut each into 4 pieces. In a medium bowl, combine Parmesan cheese, basil, parsley flakes, and garlic. Dip biscuit pieces first in Italian dressing, then in Parmesan cheese mixture. Arrange biscuit pieces in prepared pie plate. Evenly drizzle any remaining Italian dressing and Parmesan cheese mixture over top. Arrange tomatoes over biscuit pieces. Sprinkle mozzarella cheese evenly over top. Bake for 12 to 14 minutes or until biscuits are golden brown and cheese is melted. Cut into 6 wedges.

Each serving equals:

HE: 1 1/4 Bread • 1 Protein • 1/4 Vegetable • 3 Optional Calories

131 Calories • 3 gm Fat • 7 gm Protein • 19 gm Carbohydrate • 484 mg Sodium • 47 mg Calcium • 1 gm Fiber

DIABETIC: 1 Starch • 1/2 Meat

Apricot-Pecan Biscuits

Here's what I suggest: Chop the apricots and stir up the dry ingredients the night before you want to serve these delectable morning treats. Then, when you've got at least one eye open in the morning, add the liquids and combine, then bake. In no time at all, you've got fresh-baked beauties that really start the day off right!

⏺ Serves 8

> 1 cup (one 8-ounce can) apricots, packed in fruit juice, drained,
>   and ⅓ cup liquid reserved
> 1½ cups Bisquick Reduced Fat Baking Mix
> 2 tablespoons (½ ounce) chopped pecans
> 1 tablespoon Sugar Twin or Sprinkle Sweet
> ⅓ cup skim milk

Preheat oven to 375 degrees. Spray a baking sheet with butter-flavored cooking spray. Coarsely chop apricots and set aside. In a large bowl, combine baking mix, pecans, and Sugar Twin. Add reserved apricot liquid and skim milk. Mix well to combine. Stir in apricots. Drop by tablespoonful onto prepared baking sheet to form 8 biscuits. Bake for 8 to 12 minutes or until golden brown.

Each serving equals:

HE: 1 Bread • ¼ Fruit • ¼ Fat • 5 Optional Calories

119 Calories • 3 gm Fat • 2 gm Protein •
21 gm Carbohydrate • 268 mg Sodium •
35 mg Calcium • 1 gm Fiber

DIABETIC: 1 Starch • ½ Fat

Sticky Cherry Pecan Rolls

It's hard to walk through a mall these days without being overcome by the sweet scent of sticky buns, but all that sugar and fat isn't very healthy. Now you can savor my own version of sticky buns that are stuffed with fruit and nuts and really tasty! Aren't you glad you waited? ☻   Serves 8

8 Rhodes frozen yeast rolls
1 (4-serving) package JELL-O sugar-free vanilla cook-and-serve pudding mix
1 (4-serving) package JELL-O sugar-free cherry gelatin
2 cups (one 16-ounce can) tart red cherries, packed in water, drained, and ½ cup liquid reserved
¾ cup water
¼ cup (1 ounce) chopped pecans

Place rolls in a 9-by-9-inch cake pan sprayed with butter-flavored cooking spray. Cover, let thaw, and rise. Meanwhile, in a medium saucepan, combine dry pudding mix and dry gelatin. Stir in cherries, reserved cherry liquid, and water. Cook over medium heat until mixture thickens and starts to boil, stirring constantly, being careful not to crush cherries. Remove from heat. Stir in pecans. Let cool completely until rolls have risen. Spoon cooled cherry mixture between and over rolls. Cover and let set for 10 minutes. Bake at 375 degrees for 15 to 20 minutes. Place cake pan on a wire rack and allow to cool. Cut into 8 servings.

Each serving equals:

HE: 1 Bread • ½ Fruit • ½ Fat • 14 Optional Calories

164 Calories • 4 gm Fat • 5 gm Protein •
27 gm Carbohydrate • 359 mg Sodium •
8 mg Calcium • 1 gm Fiber

DIABETIC: 1 Starch • ½ Fruit • ½ Fat

Tomato Carrot Muffins

These savory muffins, piled high in a basket, are a delicious choice for your next barbecue or picnic dinner on the patio. As they bake, the Parmesan cheese melts into the batter, and hardly anything smells more delightful than that! ◐ Serves 8

1½ cups Bisquick Reduced
    Fat Baking Mix
1 teaspoon dried parsley flakes
¼ cup Sugar Twin or Sprinkle
    Sweet
¼ cup (¾ ounce) grated
    Kraft fat-free Parmesan
    cheese

6 tablespoons skim milk
2 teaspoons vegetable oil
1 egg or equivalent in egg
    substitute
¾ cup peeled and chopped
    fresh tomatoes
¼ cup finely shredded carrots

Preheat oven to 400 degrees. Spray 8 wells of a 12-hole muffin pan with butter-flavored cooking spray or line with paper liners. In a large bowl, combine baking mix, parsley flakes, Sugar Twin, and Parmesan cheese. In a small bowl, combine skim milk, vegetable oil, and egg. Add milk mixture to baking mix mixture. Mix gently just to combine. Stir in tomatoes and carrots. Evenly spoon batter into prepared muffin wells. Bake for 15 to 18 minutes or until a toothpick inserted in center comes out clean. Place muffin pan on a wire rack and allow to cool for 5 minutes. Remove muffins from pan and continue cooling on wire rack.

HINT: Fill unused muffin wells with water. It protects the muffin tin and ensures even baking.

Each serving equals:

HE: 1 Bread • ¼ Fat • ¼ Vegetable • ¼ Protein •
8 Optional Calories

115 Calories • 3 gm Fat • 3 gm Protein •
19 gm Carbohydrate • 318 mg Sodium •
38 mg Calcium • 1 gm Fiber

DIABETIC: 1 Starch • ½ Fat

Magic Morning Muffins

"Fresh from the oven" doesn't come any easier than this! Preparing these is almost as quick as opening a box of store-bought pastries—but these are so much tastier. These moist and fragrant muffins will fill the house with a wonderful aroma that's even better than an alarm clock.   ● Serves 8

> 1 cup self-rising flour
> 3 tablespoons Sugar Twin or Sprinkle Sweet
> 1/4 teaspoon apple pie spice
> 1/2 cup skim milk
> 2 tablespoons Kraft fat-free mayonnaise
> 1/2 cup raisins

Preheat oven to 425 degrees. Spray 8 wells of a 12-hole muffin pan with butter-flavored cooking spray or line with paper liners. In a medium bowl, combine flour, Sugar Twin, and apple pie spice. Add skim milk and mayonnaise. Mix well to combine. Fold in raisins. Evenly spoon batter into muffin wells. Bake for 10 to 12 minutes or until a toothpick inserted in center comes out clean. Lightly spray tops of muffins with butter-flavored cooking spray. Place muffin pan on a wire rack and let set 5 minutes. Remove muffins from pan and continue cooling on wire rack.

HINTS: 1. Fill unused muffin wells with water. It protects the muffin tin and ensures even baking.
        2. If you don't have self-rising flour, substitute with 1 cup regular flour, 1/2 teaspoon salt, and 1 1/2 teaspoons baking powder.

Each serving equals:

HE: 2/3 Bread • 1/2 Fruit • 8 Optional Calories

88 Calories • 0 gm Fat • 2 gm Protein •
20 gm Carbohydrate • 41 mg Sodium •
26 mg Calcium • 1 gm Fiber

DIABETIC: 1 Starch • 1/2 Fruit

Mandarin Almond Spice Muffins ❄

I enjoy stirring all kinds of different ingredients into muffins, just to see how a combination might work. These nutty, fruity treats taste like something your grandma might have baked for you if you were really, really good!   ◐   Serves 8

> 1½ cups all-purpose flour
> ½ cup Sugar Twin or Sprinkle Sweet
> ¼ cup (1 ounce) chopped slivered almonds
> 1 teaspoon baking soda
> 1 teaspoon baking powder
> 1 teaspoon pumpkin pie spice
> ½ cup unsweetened applesauce
> 1 egg or equivalent in egg substitute
> ¼ cup skim milk
> ½ teaspoon almond extract
> 1 cup (one 11-ounce can) mandarin oranges, rinsed, drained, and
>   chopped

Preheat oven to 400 degrees. Spray 8 wells of a 12-hole muffin pan with butter-flavored cooking spray or line with paper liners. In a large bowl, combine flour, Sugar Twin, almonds, baking soda, baking powder, and pumpkin pie spice. In a small bowl, combine applesauce, egg, skim milk, and almond extract. Add applesauce mixture to flour mixture. Mix gently just to combine. Fold in mandarin oranges. Evenly spoon batter into prepared muffin wells. Bake for 15 to 20 minutes or until a toothpick inserted in center comes out clean. Place muffin pan on a wire rack and let set 5 minutes. Remove muffins from pan and continue cooling on wire rack.

HINT: Fill unused muffin wells with water. It protects the muffin tin and ensures even baking.

Each serving equals:

HE: 1 Bread • ⅓ Fruit • ¼ Fat • ¼ Protein •
12 Optional Calories

139 Calories • 3 gm Fat • 4 gm Protein •
24 gm Carbohydrate • 233 mg Sodium •
65 mg Calcium • 1 gm Fiber

DIABETIC: 1½ Starch/Carbohydrate • ½ Fat

Robin's Walnut Waffles with Pineapple Cream Topping

Are you in a breakfast rut? Tired of spreadable fruit and a bit of fat-free cream cheese on your reduced-calorie bread? (Don't get me wrong; that's one of my standard morning meals!) Then it's time to break out and run a little wild! These creamy-topped waffles are so sweet and crunchy, you'll feel like a new person.

☻   Serves 6

> 1 cup (one 8-ounce can) crushed pineapple, packed in fruit juice, drained
> ¾ cup Cool Whip Free
> 2 tablespoons Cary's Sugar Free Maple Syrup
> 1½ cups Bisquick Reduced Fat Baking Mix
> ⅔ cup Carnation Nonfat Dry Milk Powder
> ¼ cup (1 ounce) chopped walnuts
> 1 tablespoon Sugar Twin or Sprinkle Sweet
> 1 cup water
> 1 teaspoon vanilla extract
> 1 egg or equivalent in egg substitute

In a medium bowl, combine pineapple, Cool Whip Free, and maple syrup. Cover and refrigerate while preparing waffles. In a large bowl, combine dry baking mix, dry milk powder, walnuts, and Sugar Twin. Add water, vanilla extract, and egg. Mix well to combine. Using ⅔ cup batter per serving, bake waffles according to waffle manufacturer's directions. For each serving, place 1 waffle on a plate and top with about ¼ cup pineapple mixture. Serve at once.

Each serving equals:

HE: 1⅓ Bread • ⅓ Skim Milk • ⅓ Protein • ⅓ Fat • ⅓ Fruit • ¼ Slider • 4 Optional Calories

219 Calories • 7 gm Fat • 7 gm Protein • 32 gm Carbohydrate • 390 mg Sodium • 131 mg Calcium • 1 gm Fiber

DIABETIC: 2 Starch/Carbohydrate • 1 Fat

Coconut Quick Bread

I think I was contemplating a pecan-and-coconut-topped coffeecake when I created the recipe for this rich and nutty sweet bread. If you can resist the temptation, let the bread cool thoroughly before you slice it, so the pieces won't crumble.

☺ Serves 8

> 1½ cups Bisquick Reduced Fat Baking Mix
> 1 (4-serving) package JELL-O sugar-free instant vanilla pudding mix
> ¼ cup Brown Sugar Twin☆
> 1 teaspoon baking powder
> 1 teaspoon baking soda
> ¼ cup (1 ounce) chopped pecans
> ¼ cup flaked coconut☆
> ⅓ cup Yoplait plain fat-free yogurt
> ⅓ cup Kraft fat-free mayonnaise
> ¾ cup water
> 2 teaspoons coconut extract

Preheat oven to 350 degrees. Spray a 9-by-5-inch loaf pan with butter-flavored cooking spray. In a large bowl, combine baking mix, dry pudding mix, 2 tablespoons Brown Sugar Twin, baking powder, and baking soda. Stir in pecans and 2 tablespoons coconut. In a medium bowl, combine yogurt, mayonnaise, water, and coconut extract. Add yogurt mixture to baking mix mixture. Mix gently to combine. Spread batter into prepared loaf pan. In a small bowl, combine remaining 2 tablespoons coconut and remaining 2 tablespoons Brown Sugar Twin. Evenly sprinkle topping mixture over batter. Bake for 45 to 55 minutes or until a toothpick inserted in center comes out clean. Place pan on a wire rack and let cool 5 minutes. Remove bread from pan and continue cooling on wire rack. Cut into 8 thick or 16 thin slices.

Each serving equals: (1 thick or 2 thin slices)

HE: 1 Bread • ½ Fat • ¼ Slider •
13 Optional Calories

145 Calories • 5 gm Fat • 3 gm Protein •
22 gm Carbohydrate • 697 mg Sodium •
12 mg Calcium • 0 gm Fiber

DIABETIC: 1½ Starch/Carbohydrate • ½ Fat

Apricot Banana Bread

This quick bread is so full of fruit, it's like a party in a pan! You'll be delighted to discover just how moist a bread can be when it's made with pudding *and* applesauce. ☺ Serves 8

⅔ cup Carnation Nonfat Dry
    Milk Powder
⅔ cup water
1 teaspoon white vinegar
1½ cups all-purpose flour
1 (4-serving) package
    JELL-O sugar-free
    instant banana cream
    pudding mix
¼ cup Sugar Twin or Sprinkle
    Sweet
1 teaspoon baking soda

1 teaspoon baking powder
½ cup (3 ounces) chopped
    dried apricots
¼ cup (1 ounce) chopped
    walnuts
⅔ cup (2 medium) mashed
    ripe bananas
1 egg or equivalent in egg
    substitute
½ cup unsweetened
    applesauce

Preheat oven to 350 degrees. Spray a 9-by-5-inch loaf pan with butter-flavored cooking spray. In a small bowl, combine dry milk powder, water, and vinegar. Set aside. In a large bowl, combine flour, dry pudding mix, Sugar Twin, baking soda, and baking powder. Stir in apricots and walnuts. In a medium bowl, combine bananas, egg, and applesauce. Add milk mixture to banana mixture. Mix well to combine. Spread batter into prepared loaf pan. Bake for 50 to 55 minutes or until a toothpick inserted in center comes out clean. Place pan on a wire rack and allow to cool for 5 minutes. Remove from pan. Continue cooling on wire rack. Cut into 16 inch or 8 thick slices.

Each serving equals: (2 thin or 1 thick slice)

HE: 1 Bread • 1 Fruit • ¼ Fat • ¼ Protein •
¼ Skim Milk • ¼ Slider • 4 Optional Calories

195 Calories • 3 gm Fat • 6 gm Protein •
36 gm Carbohydrate • 429 mg Sodium •
118 mg Calcium • 2 gm Fiber

DIABETIC: 1 Starch • 1 Fruit • ½ Fat

Applesauce-Raisin Muffins

If you haven't experienced the "magic" of applesauce for yourself, take it from me—it's one of the miracle ingredients in healthy cooking, and great for turning out moist baked goods every time! And if you've never baked in your microwave, here's the recipe you've been dreaming of without even knowing it. ☻ Serves 6

¾ cup Bisquick Reduced Fat Baking Mix	½ teaspoon apple pie spice
1 tablespoon Sugar Twin or Sprinkle Sweet	¼ cup raisins
	½ cup unsweetened applesauce
1 tablespoon Brown Sugar Twin	1 tablespoon skim milk
¼ teaspoon baking soda	1 egg or equivalent in egg substitute

Line a microwave muffin ring with 6 paper liners. In a medium bowl, combine baking mix, Sugar Twin, Brown Sugar Twin, baking soda, apple pie spice, and raisins. Add applesauce, skim milk, and egg. Mix well to combine. Spoon a scant ⅔ cup batter into each prepared muffin cup. Microwave on HIGH (100% power) for 1 minute. Turn muffin ring halfway. Continue microwaving on HIGH for 1½ to 2 minutes or until tops spring back when lightly touched. Remove muffins from ring and allow to cool at least 2 minutes.

HINTS:　1. 6 (one-cup) glass custard cups lined with paper liners may be used in place of muffin ring. Just be sure to arrange in a circle in microwave.
　　　　2. Wonderful served with apple butter.

Each serving equals:

HE: ⅔ Bread • ½ Fruit • 12 Optional Calories

98 Calories • 2 gm Fat • 2 gm Protein •
18 gm Carbohydrate • 240 mg Sodium •
23 mg Calcium • 1 gm Fiber

DIABETIC: 1 Starch • ½ Fruit

Hawaiian Dew Cooler

These days, when so many people prefer non-alcoholic drinks at parties, I keep getting asked to invent some festive new drinks to serve at celebrations—or just any time at all. This one has been a real crowd-pleaser with its combo of citrusy tastes (orange, pineapple, and lemony Dew). If you don't like the flavor of rum, leave the extract out. It's still a luscious blend!

◑ Serves 6 (full ¾ cup)

> 3 cups Diet Mountain Dew
> 1 cup (one 8-ounce can) crushed pineapple, packed in fruit juice, undrained
> 1 teaspoon rum extract
> 1 (4-serving) package JELL-O sugar-free orange gelatin
> 1 cup ice cubes
> 6 thin oranges slices (optional)

In a blender container, combine Diet Mountain Dew, undrained pineapple, rum extract, and dry gelatin. Cover and process on HIGH for 15 seconds. Add ice cubes. Re-cover and continue processing on HIGH until most of ice is crushed. Pour into 6 glasses. Garnish glasses with orange slices, if desired.

Each serving equals:

HE: ⅓ Fruit • 7 Optional Calories

32 Calories • 0 gm Fat • 1 gm Protein •
7 gm Carbohydrate • 49 mg Sodium •
6 mg Calcium • 0 gm Fiber

DIABETIC: ½ Fruit

Hot Spiced Cider

When the first crisp day of autumn dawns, be sure to lay in a stock of apple and orange juice so you'll be ready to stir up this steamy cider drink. It's wonderful to serve to visiting carolers or trick-or-treaters, and it's smart to keep a pot on the stove whenever company drops in.   ● Serves 12 (1 cup)

5 cups unsweetened apple juice
1 cup unsweetened orange juice
6 cups Diet Mountain Dew
¼ cup Sugar Twin or Sprinkle Sweet
2 tablespoons Brown Sugar Twin
2 teaspoons apple pie spice

In a large saucepan, combine apple juice, orange juice, and Diet Mountain Dew. Add Sugar Twin, Brown Sugar Twin, and apple pie spice. Mix well to combine. Simmer for 15 minutes, stirring occasionally.

Each serving equals:

HE: 1 Fruit • 3 Optional Calories

56 Calories • 0 gm Fat • 0 gm Protein •
14 gm Carbohydrate • 13 mg Sodium •
12 mg Calcium • 0 gm Fiber

DIABETIC: 1 Fruit

Spiced Mocha Mix

I've been experimenting with various blends of dry drink mixes because they're just so convenient. This tasty blend of coffee and chocolate, plus a little pie spice to add sparkle, will come in handy when you've been out in the cold and need something to warm you up FAST! To keep it fresh, make sure you store it tightly covered and away from sunlight. Cheers!   ☻   Serves 12

> 1 cup Carnation Nonfat Dry Milk Powder
> ¾ cup Sugar Twin or Sprinkle Sweet
> ½ cup Carnation fat-free powdered non-dairy creamer
> ⅓ cup unsweetened cocoa
> 2 tablespoons dry instant coffee crystals
> 1 teaspoon apple pie spice

In a medium bowl, combine dry milk powder, Sugar Twin, dry non-dairy creamer, and cocoa. Add coffee crystals and apple pie spice. Mix well to combine. Store in airtight container. For each serving, spoon 3 tablespoons mocha mixture into a large mug and add ¾ cup boiling water. Mix well to combine.

Each serving equals:

HE: ¼ Skim Milk • ¼ Slider • 13 Optional Calories

65 Calories • 1 gm Fat • 4 gm Protein •
10 gm Carbohydrate • 62 mg Sodium •
74 mg Calcium • 1 gm Fiber

DIABETIC: 1 Skim Milk

Celebration Menus Made Easy and Healthy

Glories of Autumn Harvest Supper

Pennsylvania Dutch Chicken Corn Soup
Stuffed Harvest Squash
Festive Cranberry Salad
Fiesta "Steak" with Corn Salsa
Frosty Pumpkin Ice Cream Pie

Home for the Holidays Evening Buffet

Turkey Chowder
Farmhouse Skillet Potatoes
Holiday Slaw
Three Cheese Strata
John's Apple Crumb Pie
Hot Spiced Cider

Love-Is-All-Around Valentine's Day Dinner

Honey Slaw Salad
Upstate Cherry Salad
Cinque Terre Shrimp Pasta
Black Forest Cheesecake

Luck of the Irish Luncheon

Baked Potato Salad
Peas with Dill
Grandma's Easter Salad
Emerald Isle Skillet
Mocha Mint Cake Dessert

Younger than Springtime Birthday Bash

Festive Spinach Dip
Fruited Party Salad
Impossible Runzas
BBQ Beef and Potato Hash
Taffy Apple Cheesecake

Hurray for Summer Potluck Picnic

Carrot-Peanut-Apple Salad
Mediterranean Macaroni Salad
Boston Baked Corn
Ranchero Meatloaf
Apricot Banana Bread
Peach Blueberry Pie

Making Healthy Exchanges Work for You

You're ready now to begin a wonderful journey to better health. In the preceding pages, you've discovered the remarkable variety of good food available to you when you begin eating the Healthy Exchanges way. You've stocked your pantry and learned many of my food preparation "secrets" that will point you on the way to delicious success.

But before I let you go, I'd like to share a few tips that I've learned while traveling toward healthier eating habits. It took me a long time to learn how to eat *smarter*. In fact, I'm still working on it. But I am getting better. For years, I could *inhale* a five-course meal in five minutes flat—and still make room for a second helping of dessert!

Now I follow certain signposts on the road that help me stay on the right path. I hope these ideas will help point you in the right direction as well.

1. **Eat slowly** so your brain has time to catch up with your tummy. Cut and chew each bite slowly. Try putting your fork down between bites. Stop eating as soon as you feel full. Crumple your napkin and throw it on top of your plate so you don't continue to eat when you are no longer hungry.

2. **Smaller plates** may help you feel more satisfied by your food portions *and* limit the amount you can put on the plate.

3. **Watch portion size.** If you are *truly* hungry, you can always add more food to your plate once you've finished your initial serving. But remember to count the additional food accordingly.

4. **Always eat at your dining-room or kitchen table.** You deserve better than nibbling from an open refrigerator or over the sink. Make an attractive place setting, even if you're eating alone. Feed your eyes as well as your stomach. By always eating at a table, you will become much more aware of your true food intake. For some reason, many of us conveniently "forget" the food we swallow while standing over the stove or munching in the car or on the run.

5. **Avoid doing anything else while you are eating.** If you read the paper or watch television while you eat, it's easy to consume too much food without realizing it, because you are concentrating on something else besides what you're eating. Then, when you look down at your plate and see that it's empty, you wonder where all the food went and why you still feel hungry.

Day by day, as you travel the path to good health, it will become easier to make the right choices, to eat *smarter*. But don't ever fool yourself into thinking that you'll be able to put your eating habits on cruise control and forget about them. Making a commitment to eat good healthy food and sticking to it takes some effort. But with all the good-tasting recipes in this Healthy Exchanges cookbook, just think how well you're going to eat—and enjoy it—from now on!

Healthy Lean Bon Appetit!

Index

I want to hear from you . . .

Besides my family, the love of my life is creating "common folk" healthy recipes and solving everyday cooking questions in *The Healthy Exchanges Way*. Everyone who uses my recipes is considered part of the Healthy Exchanges Family, so please write to me if you have any questions, comments, or suggestions. I will do my best to answer. With your support, I'll continue to stir up even more recipes and cooking tips for the Family in the years to come.

Write to: JoAnna M. Lund
              c/o Healthy Exchanges, Inc.
              P.O. Box 124
              DeWitt, IA 52742

If you prefer, you can fax me at 1-319-659-2126 or contact me via E-mail by writing to HealthyJo@aol.com. Or visit my Healthy Exchanges Internet Web site at: http://www.healthyexchanges.com.

If you're ever in the DeWitt, Iowa, area, stop in and visit me at "The House That Recipes Built" and dine at **JO's Kitchen Cafe**, "Grandma's Comfort Food Made Healthy!"

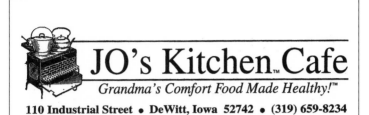

JO's Kitchen™ Cafe

Grandma's Comfort Food Made Healthy!™

110 Industrial Street • DeWitt, Iowa 52742 • (319) 659-8234

Ever since I began stirring up Healthy Exchanges recipes, I wanted every dish to be rich in flavor and lively in taste. As part of my pursuit of satisfying eating and healthy living for a lifetime, I decided to create my own line of spices.

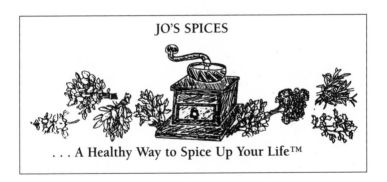

JO'S SPICES

. . . A Healthy Way to Spice Up Your Life™

JO's Spices are salt-, sugar-, wheat-, and MSG-free, and you can substitute them in any of the recipes calling for traditional spice mixes. If you're interested in hearing more about my special blends, please call Healthy Exchanges at 1-319-659-8234 for more information or to order. If you prefer, write to JO's Spices, c/o Healthy Exchanges, P.O. Box 124, DeWitt, IA 52742.

Now That You've Seen
The Arthritis Healthy Exchanges Cookbook,
Why Not Order
The Healthy Exchanges Food Newsletter?

If you enjoyed the recipes in this cookbook and would like to cook up even more of these "common folk" healthy dishes, you may want to subscribe to *The Healthy Exchanges Food Newsletter*.

This monthly 12-page newsletter contains 30-plus new recipes *every month* in such columns as:

- Reader Exchange
- Reader Requests
- Recipe Makeover
- Micro Corner
- Dinner for Two

- Crock Pot Luck
- Meatless Main
  Dishes
- Rise & Shine
- Our Small World

- Brown Bagging It
- Snack Attack
- Side Dishes
- Main Dishes
- Desserts

In addition to all the recipes, other regular features include:

- The Editor's Motivational Corner
- Dining Out Question & Answer
- Cooking Question & Answer
- New Product Alert
- Success Profiles of Winners in the Losing Game
- Exercise Advice from a Cardiac Rehab Specialist
- Nutrition Advice from a Registered Dietitian
- Positive Thought for the Month

Just as in this cookbook, all *Healthy Exchanges Food Newsletter* recipes are calculated in three distinct ways: 1) Weight Loss Choices, 2) Calories with Fat and Fiber Grams, and 3) Diabetic Exchanges.

The cost for a one-year (12-issue) subscription with a special Healthy Exchanges 3-ring binder to store the newsletters in is $28.50, or $22.50 without the binder. To order, simply complete the form and mail to us *or* call our toll-free number and pay with your VISA or MasterCard.

_____ Yes, I want to subscribe to *The Healthy Exchanges Food Newsletter.* $28.50 Yearly Subscription Cost with Storage Binder $_____

_____ $22.50 Yearly Subscription Cost without Binder . . . . $_____

_____ Foreign orders please add $6.00 for money exchange and extra postage . . . . $_____

_____ I'm not sure, so please send me a sample copy at $2.50 . . . . $_____

Please make check payable to HEALTHY EXCHANGES or pay by VISA/MasterCard

CARD NUMBER: _____ EXPIRATION DATE: _____

SIGNATURE: _____
              Signature required for all credit card orders.

Or Order Toll-Free, using your credit card, at 1-800-766-8961

NAME: _____

ADDRESS: _____

CITY: _____ STATE: _____ ZIP: _____

TELEPHONE:(   ) _____

If additional orders for the newsletter are to be sent to an address other than the one listed above, please use a separate sheet and attach to this form.

MAIL TO: **HEALTHY EXCHANGES**
          P.O. BOX 124
          DeWitt, IA 52742-0124

          1-800-766-8961 for Customer Orders
          1-319-659-8234 for Customer Service

Thank you for your order, and for choosing to become a part of the Healthy Exchanges Family!

About the Author

JoAnna M. Lund, a graduate of the University of Western Illinois, worked as a commercial insurance underwriter for eighteen years before starting her own business, Healthy Exchanges, Inc., which publishes cookbooks, a monthly newsletter, motivational booklets, and inspirational audiotapes. Her first book, **Healthy Exchanges Cookbook**, has more than 500,000 copies in print. A popular speaker with hospitals, support groups for heart patients and diabetics, and service and volunteer organizations, she has appeared on QVC, on hundreds of regional television and radio shows, and has been featured in newspapers and magazines across the country.

The recipient of numerous business awards, JoAnna was an Iowa delegate to the national White House Conference on Small Business. She is a member of the International Association of Culinary Professionals, the Society for Nutritional Education, and other professional publishing and marketing associations. She lives with her husband, Clifford, in DeWitt, Iowa.

About the Introducer

Sara B. Kramer, M.D., F.A.C.R., is a graduate of SUNY Brooklyn Medical School, a Fellow of the American College of Rheumatology, and on the faculty of New York University Medical School, where she is Assistant Professor of Clinical Medicine. In addition to her private practice in rheumatology, she is on the Board of Governors of the New York chapter of the Arthritis Foundation, where she serves on the Medical and Scientific Committee and the Patient Services Committee.

Healthy Exchanges recipes are a great way to begin—
but if your goal is living healthy for a lifetime,

You Need **HELP!**

JoAnna M. Lund's
Healthy Exchanges Lifetime Plan

"I lost 130 pounds and reclaimed my health by following a
Four Part Plan that emphasizes not only Healthy Eating, but
also Moderate Exercise, Lifestyle Changes and Goal-setting,
and most important of all, Positive Attitude."

- If you've lost weight before but failed to keep if off . . .
- If you've got diabetes, high blood pressure, high cholesterol, or heart disease—and you need to re-invent your
  lifestyle . . .
- If you want to raise a healthy family and encourage good
  lifelong habits in your kids . . .

HELP is on the way!

- The Support You Need • The Motivation You Want •
  • A Program That Works •

HELP: Healthy Exchanges Lifetime Plan
is available at your favorite bookstore

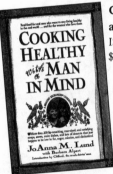
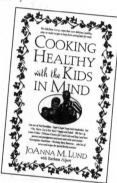
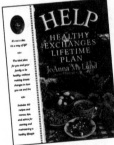
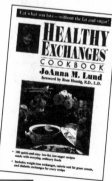